Trusted advice

Your **antenatal care**

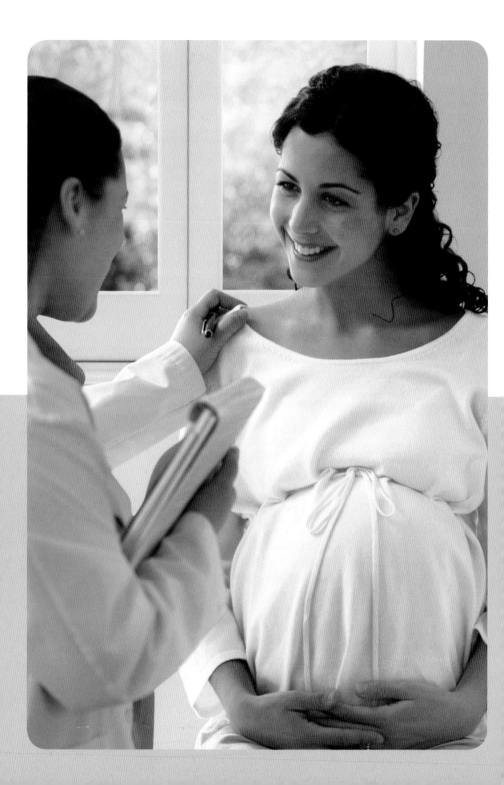

Trusted advice

Your **antenatal care**

A comprehensive guide to routine health checks
and medical care throughout pregnancy

DR**miriam**stoppard

LONDON, NEW YORK, MUNICH,
MELBOURNE, AND DELHI

Author's dedication: For Linzi

Revised Edition
Assistant Editor Dharini
Editors Bushra Ahmed, Sreshtha Bhattacharya
Assistant Designer Arijit Ganguly
Designer Anchal Kaushal
Senior Designers Tannishtha Chakraborty,
Sudakshina Basu
Managing Editor Suchismita Banerjee
Design Manager Arunesh Talapatra
DTP Operator Vishal Bhatia
DTP Designers Pushpak Tyagi, Nand Kishor Acharya
DTP Manager Sunil Sharma
Picture Researcher Sakshi Saluja

Project Editor Daniel Mills
Senior Art Editors Isabel de Cordova, Edward Kinsey
Managing Editor Penny Warren
Managing Art Editor Glenda Fisher
Publisher Peggy Vance
Senior Production Editor Jennifer Murray
Creative Technical Support Sonia Charbonnier
Senior Production Controller Man Fai Lau

First published by Dorling Kindersley in 1998

This revised edition published in Great Britain in 2012
by Dorling Kindersley Limited
80 Strand, London WC2R ORL
A Penguin Company

001–178121–02/2012
Copyright © 1998, 2012
Dorling Kindersley Limited
Text copyright © 1998, 2012
Dr Miriam Stoppard
The moral right of Miriam Stoppard to be identified
as the author of this book has been asserted.

The advice in this book is not intended as a substitute for
consultation with your healthcare provider. If you have any
concerns about the health of your baby, ask your doctor,
health visitor, or other health professional for advice.

Material in this publication was previously published by
Dorling Kindersley in Conception, Pregnancy, and Birth
by Dr Miriam Stoppard.

A CIP catalogue record for this book is available
from the British Library.

ISBN 978-1-4053-5649-7

Reproduced by Colourscan, Singapore
Printed in China by Leo Paper

Discover more at
www.dk.com

Contents

Chapter 1

Your pregnancy timetable 7

Pregnant! 8

First trimester 12

Second trimester 14

Third trimester 16

Diet in pregnancy 18

Chapter 2

Routine early care 21

Your professional carers 22

Antenatal care 24

Antenatal tests 26

Ultrasound scan 32

Chapter 3

Choosing the birth you want 35

Childbirth philosophers 36

Your choices in childbirth 38

Home or hospital? 40

Selecting a hospital 42

Preparing for a home birth 44

Childbirth classes 46

Preparation for labour 48

Fit for pregnancy 50

Your birth plan 52

Birth plan questions 54

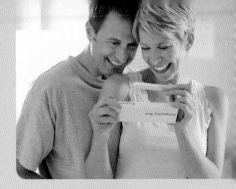

Chapter 4

Special procedures 55

Special tests 56
Rhesus incompatibility 62
Is my baby overdue? 64

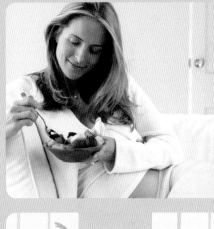

Chapter 5

Medical emergencies 67

Emergency conditions 68
Your rights 74

Useful addresses 77
Index 78
Acknowledgments 80

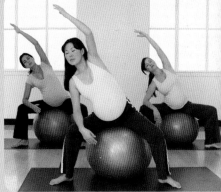

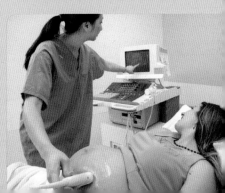

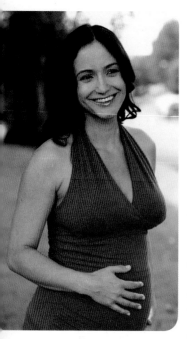

Introduction

After receiving the exciting news that you are pregnant, you'll have lots to think about and prepare: what kind of birth do you want – in hospital or at home, with medical management or as natural as possible? What are the options for pain relief? The choices are yours but it's worth looking into the various childbirth philosophies. You then need to discuss your ideas fully with your partner, doctor, and midwife. When you have decided, it's a good idea to write a birth plan so that everyone is aware of your preferences.

Attending all your antenatal check-ups is vital to protect the wellbeing of both you and your baby. At the antenatal clinic, you'll have routine tests that are designed to spot any problems and treat them promptly if necessary. Special tests, such as ultrasound scans, are offered to enable doctors to investigate the baby's health in more detail. Regular antenatal care can provide reassurance and the chance to discuss issues that you may be concerned about.

Your developing baby

For you, early pregnancy may mean that high levels of pregnancy hormones bring on nausea or sickness, the need to go to the lavatory more often, and breast tenderness. As your pregnancy becomes established, you will probably be keen to understand the developmental stages of your unborn baby, and how you can best provide good health. This means giving up smoking and avoiding alcohol, and trying to maintain a balanced diet. Keeping fit and supple in pregnancy helps your body to cope better with the extra weight; you'll also find it helps you to recover from the delivery.

Most women have normal pregnancies, but for those with existing medical conditions or an unexpected problem such as high blood pressure, it can be worrying. However, with careful monitoring and treatment, most have a successful outcome.

Chapter 1

Your pregnancy timetable

Discovering that you are pregnant for the first time can be one of the **most exciting** **moments** of your life. It's a special time, and now that a **baby is on the way,** you have to **plan and prepare for the future.**

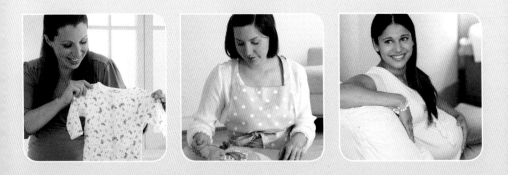

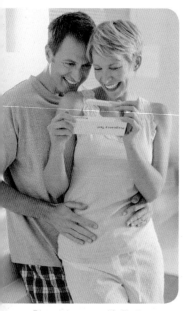

Discovering a new life Finding out you are pregnant can be one of the most special moments in your life.

Pregnant!

Many women feel that they "know" when they conceive. This special intuitive feeling is probably due to the early outpouring of female hormones, initially prolonged high levels of progesterone (which a woman does not experience unless she is pregnant), followed by human chorionic gonadotrophin (hCG) produced by the fetal tissues as soon as the embryo achieves implantation, about seven days after fertilization.

Suspecting that you are pregnant

There are certain classic signs that can make you suspect that you are pregnant before seeking confirmation. But not everybody feels the full range of pregnancy symptoms as soon as they become pregnant, and it is not uncommon for some women to experience no symptoms at all.

Amenorrhoea Within two weeks of fertilization, a woman may miss a period. Although pregnancy is the most common cause of amenorrhoea, it is not the only one, so a missed period should not be taken as an absolute sign of pregnancy. Several other factors, such as severe illness, surgery, shock, bereavement, or great stress, can also cause amenorrhoea.

Periods, however, do not always stop in pregnancy: some women have been known to have light periods up to the sixth month, and occasionally throughout their pregnancies.

Frequency of urination As soon as progesterone levels rise and the embryo starts to secrete hCG, the blood supply to the pelvic area increases, which leads to pelvic congestion. This is then communicated to the bladder, which itself becomes "irritable" and tries to expel even the smallest quantity of urine. Most women, therefore, experience the desire to urinate more frequently than usual.

Tiredness Fatigue is partly due to very high levels of progesterone, which has a sedative effect. During early pregnancy your metabolism speeds up in order to support your developing embryo and your vital organs, which have to cope with an increased amount of work. This can lead to extreme fatigue, which is sometimes so great that you just feel you have no choice but to sleep.

Odd tastes and cravings Saliva often reflects the chemical content of the blood and, with rising hormone levels, the taste within your mouth can change, often being described as metallic. This can also make certain foods taste different from normal. In fact, some flavours that you may usually enjoy (coffee is a common example) may even become intolerable.

There is no real scientific explanation for cravings, which can occasionally be for very odd things, such as coal, but they are thought to be the body's response to a deficiency in certain minerals and trace elements. Try to control cravings for inedible substances, as well as for high-calorie junk foods.

Morning sickness Most common in the morning, morning sickness can come on at any time of day especially when you do not eat often enough and your blood sugar drops as a result.

Smell Pregnancy often heightens your sense of smell and you may find that common odours, such as cooking smells, make you nauseous.

Breast changes Even at the start of pregnancy, breast changes may be quite obvious: your breasts can become quite lumpy and sore to the touch, the nipple area may become tender and sensitive, and will deepen in colour, and veins can become enlarged.

Confirming pregnancy

Once you suspect that you are pregnant you should seek confirmation as soon as possible. There are a variety of tests available. Some are more accurate than others.

Blood test This test has to be performed by your doctor and it can accurately detect the fetal hormone hCG (human chorionic gonadotrophin) in the blood as early as two weeks after conception – about the time your next period is due.

Urine test hCG can also be detected by means of a urine test. These tests are widely available and are over 95 per cent reliable. They can be performed as soon as two weeks after conception, although you will get the most reliable result if you wait a few days longer (see also p. 10).

Sharing the news with the world

You will obviously tell your partner that you are pregnant, and possibly your immediate family, as soon as you know yourself.

Doctor You should get in contact with your GP as soon as you can to discuss birth options and antenatal care.

Employer You should tell your employer before you attend your first antenatal clinic (see p. 24), which will probably be at about three months.

Friends and acquaintances Many women delay telling friends and acquaintances that they are pregnant until after the first three months. Although this is understandable, it is probably unnecessary once you have had your first scan.

Do you have the correct result?

A number of factors can affect whether your pregnancy test results are accurate.

✳ Improperly collected or stored urine can lead to errors.

✳ If the test is performed too early, the concentration of hCG will be too low to be detected. It is important to know when your period was due. Irregular or infrequent periods can affect the accuracy of the test.

✳ Some fertility drugs can change the results. Contraceptive pills, antibiotics, and painkillers should not have any effect.

✳ If the equipment used for the test is too hot, the result may be false. Urine must be at room temperature when tested.

Home testing

Many women prefer to find out whether they are pregnant in the privacy of their own homes because they can be sure of complete confidentiality. There are a variety of pregnancy testing kits available from chemists; these are simple to use and offer immediate results with an accuracy rate exceeding 95 per cent.

How the tests work All urine tests check for the presence of hCG (human chorionic gonadotrophin), the hormone manufactured by the blastocyst (fertilized egg). The two main types, the ring and the colour tests, involve mixing the chemical solution provided with a sample of your urine. The chemicals react according to the amount of hCG in your urine. The reaction is shown by a colour change in the tube or window strip, or coagulation is prevented, thereby causing the appearance of a dark ring in the tube. A third test can be performed by simply placing the absorbent part of the test strip in contact with the urine. From two weeks after conception, hCG may be detected in urine. Most kits advise using the test between one and four days after the first day of your missed period. However, if the test is negative, repeat it one week later when the hCG is more concentrated and the result will be more reliable. Most kits provide two tests for the purpose of confirmation.

Necessary precautions Follow the kit's instructions very carefully and do not use the test if it has been damaged in any way. Perform the test first thing in the morning, when the concentration of hCG in your urine is at its highest. Do not drink any liquids before the test as this will dilute the urine. If the test requires you to collect a sample of urine, catch it in a clean, soap-free container. It can be stored for up to 12 hours in the refrigerator if necessary.

Unexpected result There is the possibility that a test will show a positive result that becomes negative when repeated, and your period may start a few days later. Don't worry. Half of all conceptions do not become established pregnancies because the implanted egg fails to become established in the uterus and there is a miscarriage (possibly because of an abnormality). The test was positive because it was done before the loss of the fertilized egg. To avoid this error, do the test around the time of your first missed period. If there is a weakly positive result, repeat the test a few days later with a fresh sample.

Expected arrival date

Once you have confirmed that you are pregnant, your next question is almost certainly, "When will my baby be born?". About 266 days or 38 weeks pass between conception and birth. This is the same as 40 weeks from the start of your last menstrual period (LMP) because ovulation, and therefore conception, is normally two weeks after the start of your last period (see chart, below). You can work out the approximate date of the baby's arrival with calculations using the first day of your last period. The accuracy of this date is dependent on a regular 28-day cycle. If you have a shorter or longer menstrual cycle, your delivery date will probably differ slightly.

Your baby's arrival

The EDD (Estimated Delivery Date) is only approximate. You should not see it as the exact day that you will go into labour. A healthy pregnancy may last between 38 and 42 weeks.

How the chart works Find the first day of your last period on the chart by looking for the month in bold type, then look along the line to the actual date. The figure below it is your baby's EDD.

Your estimated date of delivery

| January | 1 | 2 | 3 | 4 | 5 | 6 | 7 | 8 | 9 | 10 | 11 | 12 | 13 | 14 | 15 | 16 | 17 | 18 | 19 | 20 | 21 | 22 | 23 | 24 | 25 | 26 | 27 | 28 | 29 | 30 | 31 |
| Oct/Nov | 8 | 9 | 10 | 11 | 12 | 13 | 14 | 15 | 16 | 17 | 18 | 19 | 20 | 21 | 22 | 23 | 24 | 25 | 26 | 27 | 28 | 29 | 30 | 31 | 1 | 2 | 3 | 4 | 5 | 6 | 7 |

| February | 1 | 2 | 3 | 4 | 5 | 6 | 7 | 8 | 9 | 10 | 11 | 12 | 13 | 14 | 15 | 16 | 17 | 18 | 19 | 20 | 21 | 22 | 23 | 24 | 25 | 26 | 27 | 28 |
| Nov/Dec | 8 | 9 | 10 | 11 | 12 | 13 | 14 | 15 | 16 | 17 | 18 | 19 | 20 | 21 | 22 | 23 | 24 | 25 | 26 | 27 | 28 | 29 | 30 | 1 | 2 | 3 | 4 | 5 |

| March | 1 | 2 | 3 | 4 | 5 | 6 | 7 | 8 | 9 | 10 | 11 | 12 | 13 | 14 | 15 | 16 | 17 | 18 | 19 | 20 | 21 | 22 | 23 | 24 | 25 | 26 | 27 | 28 | 29 | 30 | 31 |
| Dec/Jan | 6 | 7 | 8 | 9 | 10 | 11 | 12 | 13 | 14 | 15 | 16 | 17 | 18 | 19 | 20 | 21 | 22 | 23 | 24 | 25 | 26 | 27 | 28 | 29 | 30 | 31 | 1 | 2 | 3 | 4 | 5 |

| April | 1 | 2 | 3 | 4 | 5 | 6 | 7 | 8 | 9 | 10 | 11 | 12 | 13 | 14 | 15 | 16 | 17 | 18 | 19 | 20 | 21 | 22 | 23 | 24 | 25 | 26 | 27 | 28 | 29 | 30 |
| Jan/Feb | 6 | 7 | 8 | 9 | 10 | 11 | 12 | 13 | 14 | 15 | 16 | 17 | 18 | 19 | 20 | 21 | 22 | 23 | 24 | 25 | 26 | 27 | 28 | 29 | 30 | 31 | 1 | 2 | 3 | 4 |

| May | 1 | 2 | 3 | 4 | 5 | 6 | 7 | 8 | 9 | 10 | 11 | 12 | 13 | 14 | 15 | 16 | 17 | 18 | 19 | 20 | 21 | 22 | 23 | 24 | 25 | 26 | 27 | 28 | 29 | 30 | 31 |
| Feb/Mar | 5 | 6 | 7 | 8 | 9 | 10 | 11 | 12 | 13 | 14 | 15 | 16 | 17 | 18 | 19 | 20 | 21 | 22 | 23 | 24 | 25 | 26 | 27 | 28 | 1 | 2 | 3 | 4 | 5 | 6 | 7 |

| June | 1 | 2 | 3 | 4 | 5 | 6 | 7 | 8 | 9 | 10 | 11 | 12 | 13 | 14 | 15 | 16 | 17 | 18 | 19 | 20 | 21 | 22 | 23 | 24 | 25 | 26 | 27 | 28 | 29 | 30 |
| Mar/April | 8 | 9 | 10 | 11 | 12 | 13 | 14 | 15 | 16 | 17 | 18 | 19 | 20 | 21 | 22 | 23 | 24 | 25 | 26 | 27 | 28 | 29 | 30 | 31 | 1 | 2 | 3 | 4 | 5 | 6 |

| July | 1 | 2 | 3 | 4 | 5 | 6 | 7 | 8 | 9 | 10 | 11 | 12 | 13 | 14 | 15 | 16 | 17 | 18 | 19 | 20 | 21 | 22 | 23 | 24 | 25 | 26 | 27 | 28 | 29 | 30 | 31 |
| April/May | 7 | 8 | 9 | 10 | 11 | 12 | 13 | 14 | 15 | 16 | 17 | 18 | 19 | 20 | 21 | 22 | 23 | 24 | 25 | 26 | 27 | 28 | 29 | 30 | 1 | 2 | 3 | 4 | 5 | 6 | 7 |

| August | 1 | 2 | 3 | 4 | 5 | 6 | 7 | 8 | 9 | 10 | 11 | 12 | 13 | 14 | 15 | 16 | 17 | 18 | 19 | 20 | 21 | 22 | 23 | 24 | 25 | 26 | 27 | 28 | 29 | 30 | 31 |
| May/June | 8 | 9 | 10 | 11 | 12 | 13 | 14 | 15 | 16 | 17 | 18 | 19 | 20 | 21 | 22 | 23 | 24 | 25 | 26 | 27 | 28 | 29 | 30 | 31 | 1 | 2 | 3 | 4 | 5 | 6 | 7 |

| September | 1 | 2 | 3 | 4 | 5 | 6 | 7 | 8 | 9 | 10 | 11 | 12 | 13 | 14 | 15 | 16 | 17 | 18 | 19 | 20 | 21 | 22 | 23 | 24 | 25 | 26 | 27 | 28 | 29 | 30 |
| June/July | 8 | 9 | 10 | 11 | 12 | 13 | 14 | 15 | 16 | 17 | 18 | 19 | 20 | 21 | 22 | 23 | 24 | 25 | 26 | 27 | 28 | 29 | 30 | 1 | 2 | 3 | 4 | 5 | 6 | 7 |

| October | 1 | 2 | 3 | 4 | 5 | 6 | 7 | 8 | 9 | 10 | 11 | 12 | 13 | 14 | 15 | 16 | 17 | 18 | 19 | 20 | 21 | 22 | 23 | 24 | 25 | 26 | 27 | 28 | 29 | 30 | 31 |
| July/Aug | 8 | 9 | 10 | 11 | 12 | 13 | 14 | 15 | 16 | 17 | 18 | 19 | 20 | 21 | 22 | 23 | 24 | 25 | 26 | 27 | 28 | 29 | 30 | 31 | 1 | 2 | 3 | 4 | 5 | 6 | 7 |

| November | 1 | 2 | 3 | 4 | 5 | 6 | 7 | 8 | 9 | 10 | 11 | 12 | 13 | 14 | 15 | 16 | 17 | 18 | 19 | 20 | 21 | 22 | 23 | 24 | 25 | 26 | 27 | 28 | 29 | 30 |
| Aug/Sept | 8 | 9 | 10 | 11 | 12 | 13 | 14 | 15 | 16 | 17 | 18 | 19 | 20 | 21 | 22 | 23 | 24 | 25 | 26 | 27 | 28 | 29 | 30 | 1 | 2 | 3 | 4 | 5 | 6 |

| December | 1 | 2 | 3 | 4 | 5 | 6 | 7 | 8 | 9 | 10 | 11 | 12 | 13 | 14 | 15 | 16 | 17 | 18 | 19 | 20 | 21 | 22 | 23 | 24 | 25 | 26 | 27 | 28 | 29 | 30 | 31 |
| Sept/Oct | 7 | 8 | 9 | 10 | 11 | 12 | 13 | 14 | 15 | 16 | 17 | 18 | 19 | 20 | 21 | 22 | 23 | 24 | 25 | 26 | 27 | 28 | 29 | 30 | 1 | 2 | 3 | 4 | 5 | 6 | 7 |

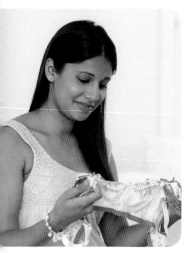

Early days In the first trimester the visible changes to your body will be slight and you will not need to buy new clothes yet. However, it may be a good idea to invest in a maternity bra early on.

First trimester

During pregnancy, the trimesters are the major milestones for the mother-to-be. Trimesters are periods of uneven length, and are defined by the rate of fetal growth rather than being simply three-month periods. By convention, the trimesters date from presumed conception (two weeks after your last period), and the first trimester represents the first 12 weeks of your baby's fetal life. The second trimester ends at 28 weeks, and the third trimester encompasses the rest of your pregnancy.

During the first trimester, your body adjusts to pregnancy. At the beginning you won't look pregnant, and you may not feel pregnant either, but the activities of your hormones will soon start to affect you in various ways. Your moods may change capriciously, your libido may decrease or increase, and you may find that your appetite changes and that you prefer blander food.

Physical changes

Your pregnant body has to work very hard to accommodate the developing embryo and the placenta. Pregnancy induces a higher metabolic rate – between 10 per cent and 25 per cent higher than normal – which means that the body accelerates all of its functions. Your heart's blood output rises steeply, almost to the maximum level that will be maintained throughout the rest of the pregnancy. Your heart rate rises, too, and will continue to do so until the middle of the second trimester. Your breathing becomes more rapid as you now send more oxygen to the fetus and exhale more carbon dioxide.

Owing to the action of oestrogen and progesterone, your breasts quickly become larger and heavier, and are usually tender to the touch from very early on. Fatty deposits are increased and new milk ducts grow. The areola around the nipple becomes darker and develops little nodules called Montgomery's tubercles. As the blood supply to the breasts increases, you will notice a network of bluish lines appearing underneath the skin.

Your uterus enlarges even in early pregnancy, but it cannot be felt through the abdominal wall until the end of the first trimester, when it begins to rise above the pelvic brim. Your uterus will increasingly press on your bladder as it enlarges, so you will need to urinate more often.

In addition, the muscle fibres of your uterus begin to thicken until it becomes very solid. However, you probably will not notice any increase in your waistline until the end of this trimester.

Taking care of yourself

You need more carbohydrates and protein to provide nutrients for your growing baby, so it is imperative that you eat healthily from the beginning of your pregnancy (see pp. 18–19). You will need more fluids, so try to drink at least eight glasses of water a day. Make sure, too, that you are getting plenty of rest. Drugs, alcohol, smoking, caffeine, and junk food should be avoided in pregnancy.

Clothes While there is probably no need to invest in maternity clothes just yet, there's nothing worse than having to put up with tight clothes and being uncomfortable, so make sure that you stay one step ahead of your increasing size. However, you are likely to need a larger support bra early on, and it should be a properly fitted maternity bra.

Your antenatal care

Your doctor may be the one who confirms your pregnancy, or you may make an appointment with the antenatal clinic as soon as you have a positive test result. If this is the case, you may not be seen until your next trimester. At the first visit, you will be asked questions about yourself, your partner, both of your families' medical histories, and your previous pregnancies (if you have had any). You will also have blood and urine tests.

Making plans

Your doctor will be able to advise you about the childbirth options available in your area. You will need to start thinking about the type of delivery you want and where you are most likely to get it. Books such as this one can help you determine your choices in childbirth as well as provide in-depth information.

You might like to start keeping a daily journal of your health and feelings during the first trimester, so that you'll have a complete record of your pregnancy. Some women feel like buying their unborn baby a little gift, such as a teddy bear, as soon as they know they're pregnant, but many feel that doing anything more than this is to tempt fate.

The early signs

Finding out that you are pregnant, especially for the first time, is extremely exciting, and you will undoubtedly long for the physical signs that will confirm the pregnancy test.

* Your breasts will grow larger, heavier, and more sensitive.

* The pigmentation of your nipples and freckles will darken.

* You may feel very tired.

* You will probably experience nausea, especially first thing in the morning.

* You will need to urinate quite frequently.

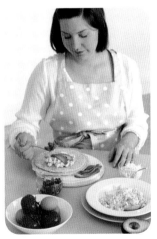

Your appetite in pregnancy Your tastes in food will change. You may experience strange tastes in your mouth, feel unusual food cravings, or entirely go off foods that you normally like.

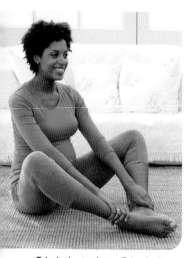

Take it slow and easy Enjoy the burst of glowing health and energy you should feel during the second trimester. Regular exercise and relaxation are beneficial during this time.

Second trimester

Now is the time when your pregnancy is well established and many of the minor complaints associated with early pregnancy have disappeared. It is also, however, the time when certain tests may need to be done. Amniocentesis (see p. 57), for example, may be offered to women with a family history of congenital abnormalities, or those with abnormal results from screening tests.

Physical changes

You may notice that your nipples begin to secrete colostrum, which is the "pre-milk" that you first feed your baby with. Your waistline will disappear and you will now "look" pregnant. Your gums may become slightly spongy, probably owing to the action of pregnancy hormones. However, there is no evidence for increased dental decay during pregnancy and absolutely no evidence to suggest that there is any truth in the saying "a tooth lost for every child".

Digestion The entire musculature of your intestinal tract is relaxed and this is the cause of many of the minor discomforts in pregnancy. Oesophageal reflux may cause heartburn because of the relaxation of the sphincter at the top of the stomach. Gastric emptying is less efficient and therefore the food remains for longer in the stomach. The relaxed intestinal muscle also leads to fewer bowel movements, and although this permits more complete absorption of foods, it can also often lead to constipation during pregnancy.

Your increasing size Generally speaking, once your uterus has expanded above your pelvis, your waistline will begin to disappear and you will need to wear larger and looser clothing. Yet the second trimester is a classic time for women to be told that they look small for their expected delivery dates. If this happens to you, don't worry.

How big you look will depend on many factors including your height and build, whether this is your first pregnancy or not (because the uterine muscle tends to get stretched after the first child), and the size of your baby, as your baby's weight increases significantly during this time. Don't compare yourself to other pregnant women – if your midwife is satisfied with the progress of your pregnancy, you should be, too.

Taking care of yourself

This is the trimester in which you will gain the most weight overall (approximately 6kg/12lb) and it is essential that you continue to eat well (see pp. 18–19). Your posture may change, as the muscles of the abdominal wall become stretched in order to accommodate your enlarging uterus. Your centre of gravity alters because you are carrying an increasing amount of weight in front. Leaning backwards may result in backache.

Backache Apart from bad posture, backache is caused by the increased blood flow to your pelvis and the rise in hormones. These cause some softening and relaxation of the ligaments of the sacroiliac joints (the sacrum), which attach your pelvic bones to your spine at the back. In addition, the ligaments and the cartilage at the front of your pelvis loosen and these joints become more mobile.

To help prevent backache, sit with your back straight and don't slouch, don't wear high-heeled shoes, and preferably sit on a hard chair or the floor. Always keep your back straight if you have to lift anything: bend from the knees and lift from a crouching position.

Your antenatal care

Regular checks of your urine, weight, and blood pressure will be made in addition to tests for chromosomal defects. During the fourth month you will have a routine ultrasound scan, and you will have the excitement of seeing your baby for the first time. You will be able to hear the incredibly fast heartbeat, and may see your baby moving.

Preparing for baby

The ideal time to prepare your baby's room and shop for baby equipment is towards the end of this trimester, when you are feeling well and full of energy. You can also begin to assemble (and have ready to pack in your hospital bag) the items you will need during labour.

Hormonal effects As the placenta takes over the production of pregnancy hormones, your hormone levels should begin to balance out. This means that you will feel more serene and positive than you did in the first trimester. Your appearance will also benefit, with thicker and shinier hair and clear and glowing skin.

Your developing pregnancy

During the second trimester you will begin to feel comfortable with being pregnant. You will enjoy the sensation of your baby moving within you and will feel energetic and full of life.

* Your libido will return or increase.

* Your abdomen will become rounded. You will lose your waistline and "look" pregnant.

* Pigmentation will continue to increase and you may notice a darker line developing down the centre of your abdomen – the *linea nigra*.

* You may suffer from indigestion and rib pain.

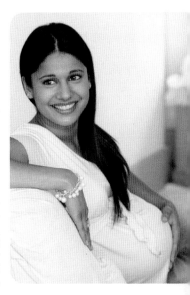

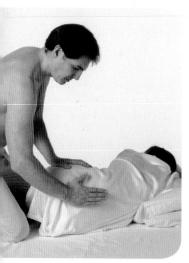

Help with relaxation If you are having trouble getting to sleep, you may find that a loving massage can help you relax.

Third trimester

You will probably feel anxious about labour and wish you could have the baby now. This doesn't mean that there is anything wrong with your baby. The sense of urgency is due to metabolic changes in the brain. Subtle shifts have gone on in each trimester, bringing about the fatigue of the first, the elation and vigour of the second, and now the anxiety and impatience of the third.

Physical changes

Your size is now increasing rapidly and you are bound to feel tired. You may find that you are not sleeping at night as well as usual and this means you will need more rest during the day. As your ligaments stretch and give way, you may find walking about increasingly uncomfortable. However, once your baby has settled into your pelvis (called engagement), you will find that your discomfort and breathlessness have diminished because the pressure on your diaphragm has been relieved.

Breathing As the baby grows bigger in the abdomen there is reduced space for the diaphragm, so pregnant women breathe more deeply and take more air in with each breath; this allows for better mixing of gases and more efficient consumption of oxygen. This has the effect of increasing the amount of air per breath from 500 millilitres to 700 millilitres (17.5 to 24.5 fluid ounces), an increase of over 40 per cent. It also means that more carbon dioxide than normal is exhaled per breath. The low level of carbon dioxide in the blood makes you feel that you are short of breath and this may be troublesome during this trimester. Relief should come when your baby engages in your pelvis and the diaphragm can once again work efficiently; your breathing rate will settle back to normal. Meanwhile, sit in a slightly propped-up position and avoid overdoing things.

Caring for yourself

As the third trimester continues, the extra weight you are carrying can result in further backache and cause you to feel continually tired. Sleep can become a problem as you get bigger, because very few positions in bed seem to be comfortable. Don't be tempted to take sleeping pills because they will make the baby sleepy, too. Take your time with everything during the last month, and make sure that you get adequate rest; catnap whenever you can and set aside periods when you can relax, even if you don't sleep. As your desire for making love may diminish or be frustrated by your increasing size, you may find that a massage can help you to relax and unwind, particularly if your partner can make it sensual. Continue to eat lots of fresh fruit and vegetables and drink at least eight glasses of fluid per day because you'll probably urinate more often. This will also help relieve constipation.

Your antenatal care

There are many tests that your midwife or doctor may use to check the baby's health or wellbeing, such as ultrasound and fetal heart rate monitoring, and your healthcare worker will discuss at each stage what is being done and why. Unlike the special tests in the second trimester – amniocentesis, chorionic villus sampling, and cordocentesis (see pp. 56–59) – none of the tests at this time are invasive of the uterus. Urine and blood pressure testing will be done frequently, as will checks for possible swelling of your feet and hands. From the 36th week until the onset of labour, you will be seen at more frequent intervals.

Preparing for the baby

Towards the end of this trimester you should have bought your baby's first clothes, sorted out the baby's room, and purchased the essential equipment. Some women stop working by the seventh month, and if you have done so, you will be able to take life at your own pace. Labour may be increasingly on your mind, and some women do find themselves worrying almost obsessively about it. Although no-one can predict exactly what will happen during your labour, because every experience is unique, be reassured that the majority of births are normal and successful.

The later months

Practical matters such as attending childbirth classes and preparing your baby's clothes and room will vie with daydreaming about the new arrival.

* You will probably get tired easily and you may find it hard to sleep at night.

* You will become increasingly aware of Braxton Hicks' contractions as your uterus practises for labour.

* You will have visited the hospital and become familiar with it and the staff. If you are having a home birth, you will have ready all the items you will need.

You may be concerned about whether you can tell if you are in labour. Even for an experienced midwife or doctor, it is difficult to know when you are in real labour. The classic signs are regular and long contractions and your waters breaking.

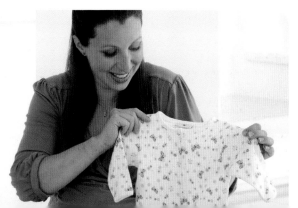

Baby's clothes and accessories You should have a selection of baby clothes, nappies, and bedding ready at least a few weeks prior to the birth.

Eating habits and nutrition

Your body will never work harder than it does during pregnancy and childbirth. To cope with the increased demands, maintain your strength, and enjoy the pregnancy, you must eat well.

Eating for you
✳ Increase your intake by 200–300 calories per day.

✳ Start to eat 5–6 small meals a day instead of 2–3 big ones.

✳ Make certain you get enough protein and carbohydrate; the former supplies essential nutrients for your developing baby and the latter meets your energy needs.

✳ Eat foods that contain vitamins, such as vitamin C, and minerals, particularly iron.

Eating for your baby
During pregnancy, you are your baby's only source of nourishment. Every calorie, vitamin, or gram of protein that your baby needs must be eaten by you. Only you can make sure that the best quality food reaches her.

Your baby needs extra protein and iron to develop well. You will fulfil all of your baby's requirements if you eat lots of fruit, green leafy vegetables, beans, peas, wholemeal cereals and pasta, fish, poultry, and low-fat dairy products. Try to eat iron-rich foods, such as red meat, eggs, raisins, apricots, and prunes.

Diet in pregnancy

Pregnant women, like most people, rarely have the time or inclination to sit around measuring out ounces of this and portions of that and trying to remember the calorific value of everything. In fact, there's no need to do that as long as you follow some basic guidelines about healthy eating in pregnancy.

One important rule is that the nearer the food is to its natural state, the more nutritious it is. So fresh food is best, frozen is next best, and you should always make tinned foods your last choice. In many ways, good nutrition is just common sense.

Eating for two?

As your pregnancy progresses your appetite will increase; this is nature's way of making certain you eat enough for you and your baby. Your energy requirements will increase only by 15 per cent, or 200–300 calories per day, far less than if you ate twice your normal amount of food. The saying "eating for two", therefore, is dangerous to follow because you'll end up putting on weight, which is extremely difficult to lose afterwards. Much more important than the quantity of what you eat is the quality. Everything you eat should be good for you and your baby. More problems develop if you eat too little rather than too much – pregnancy is not the time for dieting. It is best to balance your food intake over a 24- to 48-hour period rather than at each meal.

Daily requirements

To give you and your baby the best possible diet, try to eat the following portions each day. You should vary the food you choose:
✳ Proteins (meat, fish, eggs, cheese) – 3 servings
✳ Calcium-rich foods (cheese, milk, tinned sardines with bones) – 4 servings during pregnancy, 5 while breastfeeding
✳ Vitamin C foods (green leafy and yellow vegetables and fruit) – 3 servings
✳ Other fruit and vegetables – 1 or 2 servings
✳ Whole grains and complex carbohydrates (brown rice, wholemeal bread or pasta) – 4 or 5 servings
✳ Iron-rich food (eggs, red meat, cereals) – 2 servings
✳ Fluids – at least 8 glasses of water a day.

Essential nutrition

Eating a balanced diet is especially important during pregnancy, so make sure that your food for the day includes all the types of nourishment you and your baby need.

Carbohydrates Most of your calories should come from carbohydrates, as these are the essential fuel that gives energy. But rather than sugar-based carbohydrates, you should eat mostly complex carbohydrates in the form of wholemeal bread, porridge, brown rice, potatoes, peas, and beans and lentils, which provide long-lasting energy and fibre. Avoid processed carbohydrates such as refined sugar where possible. However, simple carbohydrates are absorbed by the system in minutes, so the sugars from fructose (fruit), lactose (milk), and dextrose (honey) are good for a quick energy boost and can help to relieve morning sickness.

Protein Proteins are the building blocks that enable all your baby's tissues – bone, muscle, cartilage, and blood – to grow, so you should eat at least 100 grams (4 ounces) of protein a day if you can. You may not necessarily eat red meat very often (or at all), but in pregnancy it is important because red meat is the most concentrated source of iron (see p. 20). For vegetarians, milk (skimmed), yogurt, cheese, and eggs are excellent sources of protein; so is the vegetable protein in seeds, nuts, peanut butter (though calorific), as well as in peas, beans, and lentils. Most bread is protein-enriched. Eat as much fish as you can – it's easily digested pure protein and rich in minerals and vitamins. Oily fish also contains essential fatty acids.

Vitamins All the vitamins are important for maintaining general good health, but some vitamins, such as B and C, cannot be stored by the body, and a daily intake is required. B vitamins are supplied in some vegetables and fruit and are also found in meat, fish, dairy products, grains, and nuts. Vitamin C is provided by fresh fruit and vegetables. Vitamin D is found in fish oils, and can be manufactured by the body if it is triggered by the action of sunlight on the skin; most people in the UK require about 40 minutes of sun per day to produce adequate amounts. Folic acid is important in the prevention of spina bifida and supplements should be taken for three months before you get pregnant and during the first trimester. Avoid liver and liver pâtés because they are high in vitamin A, which can cause problems in pregnancy.

Your weight gain

Doctors recommend that a woman of average weight, experiencing an average pregnancy, ought to gain an average of 10–13kg (22–28lb) in the total 40 weeks' gestation. This allows about 3–4kg (6–8lb) for the baby and about 7–9kg (15–20lb) for the baby's support system (comprising placenta, amniotic fluid, and increased blood, fluid, fat, and breast tissue).

* During the first trimester you will probably gain very little weight, about 1–2kg (2–4lb), if nausea hasn't been a problem. Of this, only 48g (1.7oz) will be your baby. The rest is made up of the baby's support system.

* During the second trimester, you will probably gain approximately 6kg (12lb). Of this, only 1kg (2lb) will actually be your baby. The rest is made up of the baby's support system.

* During the third trimester you will probably gain about 5kg (10lb). Of this, approximately 3–4kg (6–8lb) will be accounted for by your baby. The rest is made up of the baby's support system.

A steady gain like this means that your body can adapt more easily to your increasing size; if you are eating regularly, your baby has a continuous flow of nourishment.

Preparing healthy food

Try to develop some good cooking habits that will promote a healthy eating style.

✳ Trim the fat from meat before cooking.

✳ Skim the fat off the surface of casseroles and soups.

✳ Bake, steam, microwave, or grill rather than fry.

✳ Stir-fry in a teaspoon of olive oil, or simmer with a stock cube dissolved in a cup of water.

✳ Use non-stick pans and a minimum of fat when cooking.

✳ Add dried skimmed milk to milky drinks for extra calcium.

✳ Always choose low-fat (not full-fat) dairy products.

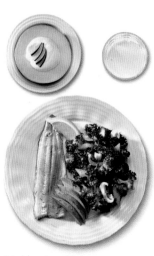

A balanced meal Salmon or trout and salad, with melon, yogurt, and nectarine to follow, and a glass of milk make a nutritious meal.

Minerals These are essential for your body to function efficiently. As soon as you conceive, calcium is needed to build your baby's skeleton and teeth. Keep your calcium intake high by including broccoli, dried milk, and tinned salmon with bones in your diet. Green leafy vegetables and dairy products also contain calcium. Remember that vitamin D is needed to promote calcium absorption.

Iron This is vital, not just for your baby but for your own needs, too. Your baby uses iron so fast that he could be said to be in a constant iron-deficient state. If you are iron-deficient when you get pregnant, or become so later on, your doctor will prescribe iron tablets or injections to prevent you from developing anaemia. Eat plenty of foods that are rich in iron, such as red meat, eggs, apricots, raisins, and prunes, but avoid liver.

Vegetarian diets

If you do not eat meat, you need to make sure you get enough protein, vitamins, and iron from other sources to meet your own and your baby's needs. Animal products also provide calcium and vitamins B_6, B_{12}, and D, which are essential for health; vitamin B_{12} supplements may be necessary if you eat no animal products.

What to avoid

Certain common precautions should be taken because we now know that some foods are contaminated with enough bacteria to cause illness, and may even cause miscarriage or birth defects.

Listeria is a rare bacterium found in soft cheese, unpasteurized milk, ready-made coleslaw, cooked chilled foods, pâtés, and improperly cooked meat. Bacteria are normally destroyed at pasteurizing temperatures, but if food is infected and refrigerated, the bacteria may continue to multiply. Avoid risky foods and wash your hands after any direct contact with animals such as sheep.

Salmonella is a bacterium found in eggs and chicken that causes fever, abdominal pain, and severe diarrhoea. It is killed by thorough cooking.

Toxoplasmosis is caused by a parasite found in cat and dog faeces and also in raw meat. It can cause birth defects. Always wash your hands after handling a pet or its litter tray and wear gloves when gardening.

Chapter 2

Routine early care

Good antenatal care makes **healthy mothers and babies**. Routine tests can spot **problems** as soon as they arise, while **special tests** are available for mothers and babies with **particular needs**.

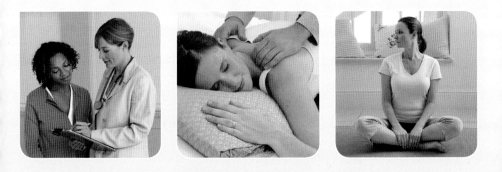

Your professional carers

There are a number of options open to you regarding who attends to your labour – it does not have to be a straight choice between hospital expertise or a home midwife. Wherever you decide to have your baby, the system can usually be tailored to suit your individual needs. Of course, the professional attendant is not the only one you should think about. Many women are supported by their partners or a friend during childbirth, and most hospitals now welcome this.

Your own GP

Your general practitioner will probably be the first professional person that you see. You need to establish his or her views on birth – especially if you are interested in having a home birth. A few doctors are happy to attend a home delivery of a normal pregnancy, many are not so willing, and some fall somewhere in between – preferring you to have had at least one straightforward delivery in hospital first.

Many doctors provide antenatal care if you are having the baby in the hospital to which they have referred you. Occasionally, you may be able to attend your doctor's clinic even if you are booked into another hospital – try to explore all of the options.

Consultant obstetricians

An obstetrician is a consultant who specializes in medical problems to do with pregnancy and childbirth. When you book into a hospital you will be assigned to an obstetrician who is part of a midwifery and medical team. You can ask to be referred to a particular obstetrician, although they may be linked to specific geographical areas.

If you feel strongly that you want a woman obstetrician, check with your hospital. If they have one, you should make your preference clear on your birth plan, although the consultant is not obliged to take you on. There is no guarantee, however, that the obstetrician of your choice will be on duty when you go into labour.

You will be unlikely to see your consultant unless you have problems in your pregnancy. Most routine medical care is provided by junior doctors working alongside midwives in the obstetrics team.

Midwives

The modern, professional midwife is a specialist in childbirth, qualified to take responsibility for you before, during, and after the birth. She is able to support and understand you during labour and delivery, and knows when to call for obstetric advice and assistance. Unlike the obstetrician, her focus is on the normal, not the abnormal. Midwives working outside hospitals tend to be more accepting of a variety of approaches than hospital carers.

Team midwives Midwives who are a part of the team midwife scheme provide a more personal service. One midwife or a team of midwives is allocated to you, and a midwife may come to your house for antenatal care, and go with you to the hospital to deliver your baby when labour starts; the hospital staff are only rarely involved. If all goes well, you are usually discharged from hospital within a few hours of the birth into her care.

Independent midwives These midwives provide continuous care in a variety of situations. They will deliver your baby wherever you choose, whether at home or in hospital, and undertake to be with you throughout the labour and delivery (see also column, right).

Hospital midwives Some midwives choose to stay within the hospital and don't go into the community. They often have senior roles on the antenatal or postnatal wards, or on the labour ward.

Independent midwives

Because your midwife will be your primary caregiver you will need to get to know her well. You may like to ask her the following questions:

✻ What experience has she had?

✻ Does she work alone or with other midwives? Will you be able to meet them?

✻ What are her considerations in managing labour?

✻ What is her back-up system? Does she work closely with any particular doctors?

✻ What equipment, drugs, and resuscitation equipment for the baby does she carry?

✻ What antenatal care does she provide? Are there home visits?

✻ Under what conditions would she transfer you to hospital?

✻ What is her fee?

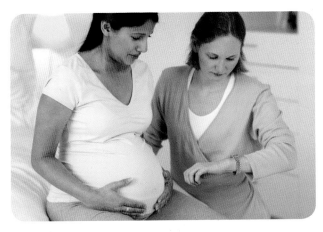

You and your baby's welfare
Your midwife will be in charge of your welfare throughout your pregnancy. The midwife or doctor will monitor the progress of your pregnancy and record details of routine tests.

Breech presentation

Most babies are born head first, but your baby may present bottom down as you go into labour – this is known as breech presentation. Four out of every 100 babies are born in this position, so it's not that unusual.

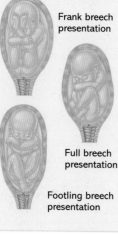

Frank breech presentation

Full breech presentation

Footling breech presentation

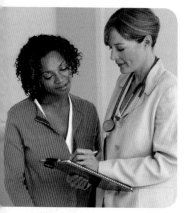

Discussing your pregnancy Don't be afraid to ask questions about what is said to you at the clinic.

Antenatal care

Although most pregnancies proceed normally, consultations, check-ups, and tests are carried out regularly to ensure a healthy pregnancy. These visits and investigations are vital to monitor your progress and spot problems before any harm is done.

The antenatal clinic

You will attend an antenatal clinic at either the hospital where you will have your baby or at your doctor's surgery. Most women attend these once a month up until week 32, then every two weeks up to 36 weeks, and then once a week for the last month. You will need to have check-ups more frequently if any complications develop.

It can be quite intimidating and frustrating to attend an antenatal clinic in a large hospital at first: there are a large number of staff coming and going, and you may often have to wait for your turn. Negative feelings can be made much worse by the discontinuity of care – it's quite possible that you will see different midwives and doctors at every visit. Such hassles can be avoided if you opt for shared care, where you mainly see your GP or your midwife for check-ups with occasional visits to the hospital clinic.

Try to make the best of your time at the antenatal clinic by taking along a book or something to keep you occupied, and some food in case you feel hungry while you are there. Take a friend or your partner with you for company and support. If you already have children, try and arrange for them to be looked after.

Talking to your carers

Antenatal clinic visits may not offer sufficient time for mothers to talk to their carers. However, discussing the alternatives open to you and your preferences, as well as being reassured about any fears and concerns you may have, is very important. So be prepared to speak up for yourself and insist on extra time if required. If you have strong preferences but worry that you won't be able to stand up for yourself, take your partner along for moral support. It will probably help if you make a list of issues beforehand.

Your file

At your first antenatal visit all the details of your past medical and obstetric (if any) history, including your menstrual history, will be noted in your file or booklet. This file contains all the details relevant to your care. Carry it with you on every visit, so that even if your carers change, the contents can be transferred from one set of case notes to the other. In addition, remember to take your file with you to the hospital when you go into labour. The details may initially be difficult to understand because many of the medical terms are abbreviated. Compare the abbreviations on your file or booklet with those that are explained below. If it still does not seem to make much sense, don't hesitate to ask your midwife or doctor.

Medical terms and abbreviations

NAD or **nil** or **a tick** No abnormality detected

Alb Albumin in urine (a name for one of the proteins found in the urine sample)

BP Blood pressure

FH Fetal heart

FHH/NH Fetal heart heard or not heard

FMF Fetal movements felt

Ceph. Cephalic, baby is head down

Vx Vertex, baby is head down

Br Breech, baby is bottom down

Long L Longitudinal lie, the baby is lying parallel to your spine in the uterus

VBAC Vaginal birth after Caesarean

LMP Last menstrual period

EDD/EDC Estimated date of delivery/confinement

Hb Haemoglobin levels, to check for anaemia

Eng/E Engaged – the baby's head has dropped down into the pelvis

NE Not engaged

Fe Iron has been prescribed

TCA To come again

Height of fundus The height of the top of the uterus. The baby pushes this up as it grows and often the height is used to estimate the length of the pregnancy. Some clinics measure the height of the fundus with a tape measure in centimetres

Relation of PP to brim This is the brim of your pelvis. The part of the baby presenting to the brim (presenting part, or PP) in the later stages of your pregnancy will be the part to be born first

PET Pre-eclamptic toxaemia

Oed Oedema

AFP Alpha-fetoprotein

CS Caesarean section

H/T Hypertension (high blood pressure)

MSU Midstream urine

Primigravida This is your first pregnancy

Multigravida You have had more than one pregnancy

VE Vaginal examination

The lie of your baby

Certain abbreviations describe how the baby is lying and refer to where the back of the baby's head (occiput) is in relation to your body – on the right or left, to the front (anterior) or back (posterior). ROA, for example, means that the back of his head is to the front on your right.

The baby's presentation will affect your labour: the posterior position may slow it down, for example.

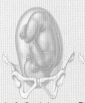

Left Occipito-Anterior (LOA)   Right Occipito-Anterior (ROA)

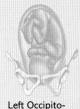

Left Occipito-Posterior (LOP)   Right Occipito-Posterior (ROP)

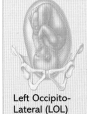

Left Occipito-Lateral (LOL)   Right Occipito-Lateral (ROL)

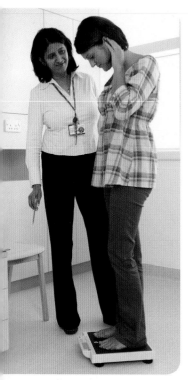

Recording your weight Details of your weight and height are recorded as part of your personal history. You will also be asked about smoking, drinking, and street drugs.

Antenatal tests

Every pregnant woman undergoes certain routine tests to keep a check on her health and the development of her baby; these may be performed at every visit or at different times during her pregnancy. Some are performed only once. If the tests indicate that there is, or that there may be, a problem, you will be monitored closely and prompt action will be taken if necessary.

Height and shoe size
Your height and shoe size will be noted at your first visit. If you are petite with small feet, you may have a small pelvis, which can affect labour. However, the chances are that your baby will be tailored to your physical build and labour will be straightforward.

Weight
In the first trimester a loss of weight is sometimes brought about by nausea and vomiting due to morning sickness, but is usually nothing to worry about. Sudden weight gain may reflect fluid retention and possibly pre-eclampsia (see p. 72).

In the past, maternal weight gain was taken as a reliable indicator of the growth of the baby. Research now indicates, however, that maternal weight gain should not be relied upon on its own, but should be viewed in conjunction with external and internal examinations, blood and urine tests, blood pressure, and ultrasound scans, as these are much more accurate in measuring fetal growth.

Legs and hands
At every visit your legs will be checked for varicose veins, and your ankles and hands will be examined for excessive swelling and puffiness (oedema). A little swelling in the final weeks of pregnancy is normal, particularly in the evening and during hot weather. Excessive or sudden swelling does, however, need investigation.

Breasts
Your breasts will be examined and the condition of your nipples will be noted. A few women have dimpled, or inverted, nipples, and these may have to be corrected by wearing a breast shield inside your bra.

Urine

At your first visit and every subsequent visit, a sample of midstream urine (obtained by passing the first few drops into the toilet bowl and collecting a sample of the midstream urine in a sterile container) will be taken to test for the presence of protein, which may be a sign of a urinary or kidney infection; for sugar, to check that you are not developing diabetes; and for ketones, which may be a sign that you are not eating properly or that your body is not metabolizing food in the correct manner. Urine testing in pregnancy can also unmask underlying diabetes. A large amount of protein in your urine in late pregnancy is a strong indication of pre-eclampsia. This will be treated promptly because of the associated potential for a growth-restricted baby or premature delivery.

Blood tests

At your first visit, a routine blood sample will be taken from a vein in your arm to find out your basic blood group (O, A, B, AB), and your Rhesus (Rh) blood group (positive or negative), in case a blood transfusion becomes necessary. If you are Rh negative, you will be tested for Rhesus incompatibility (see p. 62). Your haemoglobin level is also ascertained. This is a measure of the oxygen-carrying power of your red blood cells. The normal level is 12–14 grams; if it falls below 10 grams, treatment for anaemia is given. Iron and folic acid raise the oxygen-carrying power of blood and prevent anaemia, so make sure you eat iron-rich foods and take folic acid supplements as directed by your doctor. Further routine and special blood tests may also be carried out (see pp. 30–31).

Baby's head size and your pelvis

The shape and size of your pelvis is important because of the risk of disproportion, which could become apparent during labour and may delay the baby's delivery.

Disproportion means that your pelvis is too small for your baby's head to pass through it easily, or your baby's head is too large. To avoid delays in delivering your baby, it is important for your doctor or midwife to make an assessment of the size of your pelvic outlet. Your height and shoe size are good guides; short women who have small feet also tend to have small pelvises.

If difficulties are suspected, your baby's head size will be determined using ultrasound (see p. 32). Severe disproportion may mean delivering the baby by Caesarean section.

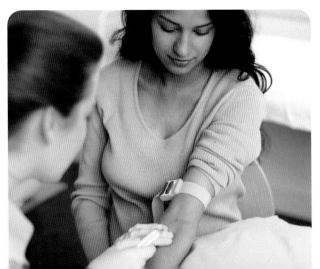

Blood is taken for tests The composition of your blood and the substances found in it may indicate actual or potential problems.

External examination

At every visit your abdomen will be palpated (felt) to determine the size of the growing baby. This will give the doctor or midwife a good idea as to whether your baby is approximately the right size for your dates and whether he is growing well. A series of measurements is taken over the course of your pregnancy that gives a very accurate picture of your baby's rate of progress. A measurement is taken of the distance between your pelvic bone and the top of your uterus (fundus), which normally enlarges into your abdomen at 14 weeks and continues until just prior to term.

The amount of amniotic fluid, as well as your individual size and weight, can have an effect on the size of your baby, so after 26–28 weeks the doctor or midwife will also feel for your baby's "poles" (head and rump). This allows them to judge the lie of your baby (see p. 25).

Internal examination

By no means will everyone have an internal examination at their first antenatal visit, but if it is carried out, the doctor or midwife will be able to confirm the pregnancy dates, check your cervix, and if necessary assess your pelvic size.

If an internal examination is to be performed, you will be asked to lie down and raise your knees. The doctor or midwife will insert two gloved fingers of one hand into your vagina and press your abdomen with the other hand to check

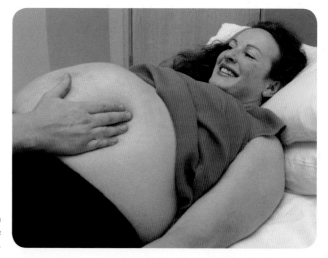

External examination Your abdomen will be felt at every visit to check the growth and position of the fetus.

the size of your uterus, to establish whether it is the right size for your dates. As long as you relax, an internal examination is usually only slightly uncomfortable. It will not harm your baby.

If at any time during your pregnancy the baby does not seem to be growing as expected, you will usually have an ultrasound to check this (see p. 32). If you experience painful contractions early on in the pregnancy or have a history of recurrent miscarriages, your cervix will be examined to see if it is tightly closed. If there is any suspicion of a weak or shortening cervix, the length can be assessed by ultrasound scanning. Further internal examinations will be carried out once labour has started.

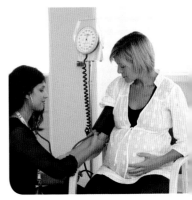

Blood pressure Your blood pressure is taken at every antenatal check and it is a significant measure of how your body is coping with the pregnancy.

Blood pressure

This reading is taken at every visit, and measures the pressure at which your heart is pumping blood through your body. The reading is made up of two figures: the upper one is the systolic pressure – when the heart contracts it pushes out blood and "beats". This is measured when the arm band is tight. As the pressure is released, the lower, or diastolic, reading is taken – this is the resting pressure between beats.

The average reading in pregnancy is 120 over 70. Blood pressure varies, however, according to your age, and there is a range of blood pressures that is considered normal for each age group. A higher reading than normal may indicate a risk of pre-eclampsia and bed-rest in hospital might be advised. Regular antenatal checks ensure that any changes are quickly noted.

Fetal heartbeat

Your baby's heartbeat will be monitored at every visit from week 24 onwards. The doctor or midwife may use a Sonicaid to listen. This small portable instrument uses ultrasound waves and is placed on your stomach. It magnifies the sound of your baby's heartbeat so that both the midwife and you can listen to it. The baby's heartbeat is almost twice as fast as your own.

Routine blood tests

You will have routine blood tests at your first antenatal visit to establish your blood group and your haemoglobin levels, and to see whether certain conditions are present. If problems are detected, you will have further, more specific blood tests.

Blood group and Rhesus (Rh) status Your doctor needs to know which blood group you belong to (A, B, O, AB) in the event of you needing a blood transfusion during the pregnancy or labour. Your Rhesus status is either negative or positive, so that you may be A negative or O positive, and so on.

If you are Rhesus negative, a further test will be performed to check for the presence of antibodies; tests are repeated at intervals during your pregnancy (see pp. 62–63). Your partner may also have to have a blood test.

Haemoglobin levels The red cells in the blood contain iron and carry oxygen; if the test shows that the number of red cells is low, or that they are short of iron, you will be advised to eat iron-rich foods or take iron tablets.

Rubella (German measles) This blood test shows whether you have developed immunity to the disease. If not, you will be at risk of contracting rubella in early pregnancy, which could cause heart defects, blindness, and deafness in the baby.

Syphilis This sexually transmitted disease is rare these days and can be easily cured. If you have the disease and it is not treated during pregnancy, it could cause serious developmental or congenital problems in your baby.

Hepatitis B This liver disease is caused by a virus. It can be passed to the baby and cause serious liver damage.

Toxoplasmosis You can also ask to have your blood tested for toxoplasmosis. The toxoplasma is a parasite that can be picked up from cat faeces and from poorly cooked meat. Toxoplasmosis is harmless to adults, but it can cross the placenta and cause blindness, epilepsy, and developmental delay in the baby. Ask for the test if you're worried, particularly if you have pets that hunt outside.

Special blood tests
Triple test (for Down's syndrome) It depends on the hospital's policy, but this test is now usually offered to all women. It shows the level of three substances in the mother's bloodstream: alpha-fetoprotein (AFP) (see column, right), oestriol, and human chorionic gonadotrophin (hCG). Abnormal

concentrations may be linked to certain fetal abnormalities. Increasingly this blood test is combined with an early scan to measure the thickness of a fold of skin at the back of the fetus' neck (see nuchal scan, p. 34).

However, a positive result in this test merely means that you have an increased risk of a Down's baby. To diagnose this or rule it out, you need further tests such as an amniocentesis (see p. 57).

Glucose tolerance test (for diabetes) This test is necessary if you have high blood sugar, sugar in the urine, a large baby, or if you've had diabetes in a previous pregnancy.

The test involves having a sugary drink, after which a sample of blood is taken two hours later. If your blood-sugar level remains high, it may indicate diabetes.

Treatment includes strict control of your diet, possibly also with insulin injections, and extra antenatal check-ups. You may also be required to have more than the usual two ultrasound scans.

HIV test (for human immunodeficiency virus) This is now offered to all pregnant women but is carried out only with your consent. If you have the disease, anti-viral treatment will be offered. The risk of transmitting HIV to your baby can be reduced by taking certain precautions at birth, and avoiding breastfeeding.

Sickle cell test (for sickle cell anaemia) This test is necessary if you, or any of your ancestors, come from an area where sickle cell anaemia is widespread, especially Africa and the West Indies.

The test examines the type of haemoglobin in your red blood cells and detects sickle-shaped cells. If sickle cell trait or disease is found, your partner should be tested as well. If he is positive, the baby is at risk of being born with the disease. An amniocentesis or cordocentesis test will confirm or rule out this possibility (see pp. 56–57).

Haemoglobin electrophoresis test (for thalassaemia)
This test is advisable if you, or any of your ancestors, come from the Mediterranean, Asia, and parts of Africa. It identifies the different haemoglobins causing thalassaemia disease. If both parents have partial abnormalities, the baby has a 1 in 4 chance of developing the disease. Amniocentesis or cordocentesis may be carried out for confirmation.

Alpha-fetoprotein

This is a protein that is first produced by part of the embryo, and then later by the fetal liver. It may be used as an indicator of what is going on inside the uterus.

AFP is commonly found in varying amounts in your blood throughout pregnancy. An abnormally low level of alpha-fetoprotein can suggest that the fetus may have Down's syndrome and you will be offered amniocentesis to confirm or rule out this diagnosis. The levels may be unusually raised because of a multiple pregnancy, inaccurate dating of the pregnancy, abnormalities of the baby's kidneys, digestive, or neurological systems, or if there is a threat of miscarriage.

Therefore, an ultrasound scan (see p. 32) will be performed to check for a multiple pregnancy, to confirm your dates in case your pregnancy is more advanced than you think, and to check the physical make-up of your baby.

Why a scan is offered

Scans are normally offered to check the baby's progress, but there are other occasions when an ultrasound scan will be useful:

✳ During infertility treatments such as IVF.

✳ To identify abnormal conditions such as an ectopic pregnancy.

✳ If the doctors suspect an imminent miscarriage.

✳ To check for a multiple pregnancy.

Ultrasound scan

With the aid of an ultrasound scan you can see a picture of your unborn baby. An ultrasound scan checks the baby's physical structure, general wellbeing, and position, and guides doctors when performing special tests and operations. You will be offered at least two scans during your pregnancy. The first is routinely performed between 10 and 14 weeks, and the second between 20 and 22 weeks. If any problems are detected, repeat scans may be performed several times before the birth.

How it works

The process is based on a sonar device that reveals objects in fluid, first used by the British navy to detect submarines during World War II. A crystal inside a device called a transducer converts an electrical current into high-frequency soundwaves that are inaudible to the human ear. The soundwaves form a beam that penetrates the abdomen as the transducer is moved back and forth. The beam reflects off material in its path, and the transducer records these echoes. The echoes are converted into electrical signals, which produce an image that can be displayed on a television-like screen. The beam can only penetrate fluids and soft tissue such as the amniotic sac, kidneys, and liver. It cannot pass through bone or register gas. An ultrasound scan is increasingly used to assess threatened miscarriage; to exclude ectopic pregnancies; during infertility treatments, such as IVF; and during fetal surgery.

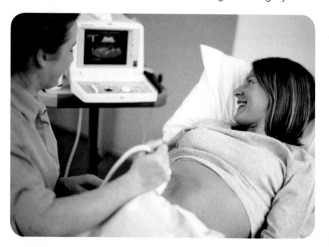

What you can see As the transducer is moved over your abdomen, the operator will explain the image on the screen.

What happens

Having a scan is painless, and usually lasts about 15 minutes. You may be asked to drink about half a litre (a pint) of water and not to urinate before arriving at the clinic. This can be uncomfortable, but a full bladder will provide a clearer picture of your baby. You may be asked to remove some clothes and put on a hospital robe before lying on a bed beside the scanner. As the transducer is passed over your abdomen, the image appears on the screen, and you can enjoy your first view of your baby.

Is it safe?

Unlike an X-ray, ultrasound scanning poses no known risk to the fetus. Questions have been raised about long-term effects, such as hearing impairment, caused by the impact of soundwaves. However, recent research seems to indicate that ultrasound is not harmful to the mother or the baby, because the waves are of a very low intensity, and so it is safe for the scan to be performed repeatedly. But if you are worried, do not have one unless it is necessary.

Your first scan

The sophisticated equipment used for an ultrasound scan may at first appear rather daunting, but don't be intimidated. The scan offers an exciting opportunity for you and your partner to see your baby for the very first time. The ultrasound operator will explain the image on the screen, but remember that scanning requires a lot of concentration and the

What it shows about your baby

A routine scan shows whether your baby is healthy, and it may be used for other reasons during your pregnancy:

✳ To check the location and development of the placenta.

✳ To check on the growth rate of the baby, particularly when the date of conception is uncertain.

✳ To discover if the baby is ready to be born, if overdue.

✳ To confirm that your baby is in the usual head-down position, and not bottom-down, after week 38.

✳ To exclude certain fetal abnormalities, such as spina bifida.

✳ To assist in any operations performed on the baby while still in the uterus.

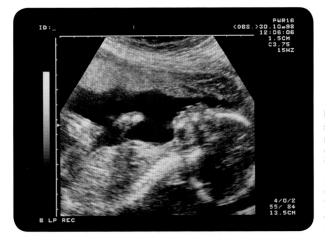

Baby at 22 weeks An ultrasound scan will clearly show your baby's shape, his position, and whether you are expecting more than one. This image shows the baby in his mother's uterus. The baby floats and moves about continuously in the amniotic sac performing various activities: sucking his thumb, yawning, blinking, hiccupping, and urinating.

Nuchal scan

This scan is of a fetus with a normal nuchal pad. The red line indicates where the neck pad would be thicker in a baby that is likely to have Down's syndrome, heart defects, or chromosomal abnormalities.

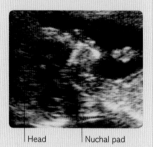

| Head | Nuchal pad |

ultrasonographer may wait until the end of the scan to talk to you. Many clinics will give you a print of the image of your baby but you may be asked to pay a small fee for this. During your first scan (usually between 10 and 14 weeks) the size and number of features will be measured, as will the baby's heartbeat and the nuchal thickness – the thickness of a pad at the back of the baby's neck (nuchal means neck). In a Down's syndrome baby, this neck pad is thicker than normal. An amniocentesis may be offered to confirm or rule out Down's syndrome and other chromosomal abnormalities.

Specialized scans

Anomaly scan You will also be offered a detailed scan of all of your baby's physical structures at 20–22 weeks. During this scan all of the baby's anatomy is checked as well as the location of the placenta. You should be able to hear the baby's heartbeat, and distinguish kicking and the gentle movement of hands and feet waving. You may be asked to come back to repeat the scan if the scanner does not pick up the baby properly.

Doppler scan This scan uses high-frequency sound waves of a different kind from those used in ordinary ultrasound scans. These are processed to reveal special wave forms, which can be used to show tiny movements within the growing fetus or placenta – for example, how the blood is moving along the main vessels. This type of scan allows the scanner operator to see whether the placenta is working as it should, or if there is a possibility that the baby is not getting enough oxygen.

Chapter 3

Choosing the birth you want

There are **many decisions** to make about the kind of labour and birth you want. A birth plan is useful, and **childbirth classes** will provide you and your partner with **practical training** and **moral support**.

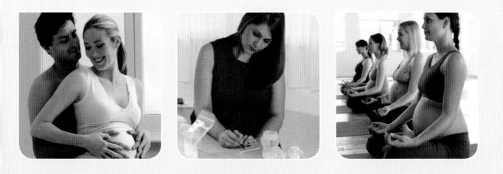

The Bradley method

This refinement of birth preparation was initiated by Dr Robert Bradley, and is also known as husband-coached childbirth.

The Bradley method teaches women to accept the pain and go with the flow, under the guidance of the husband or partner, friend, or counsellor. The coach attends the antenatal classes with the mother, helps her with her exercise and breathing routine, and comforts, coaxes, and coaches her through labour and delivery.

The failing of this method is that most women need to be distracted from pain in order to focus outside of themselves. Getting in touch with the pain can be totally overwhelming, making it harder, not easier, to cope.

Each labour is completely unpredictable and your experience may be dissimilar to what you yourself have prepared for. A woman often reacts to giving birth very differently from how she imagined. Also, some birth partners can become so enthusiastic about their coaching that they lose sight of the woman and her particular needs.

Childbirth philosophers

There have been a number of people who have influenced the way women and their carers approach birth today. Their teaching and ideas have altered antenatal and postnatal care, making childbirth an ever-evolving experience, and they have greatly affected the approach and procedures employed in childbirth in the West today. Most of these theories encourage the woman to follow her body's lead in a loving and intimate environment.

Dr Grantley Dick-Read

In the early 20th century, Dr Dick-Read was the first obstetrician to realize that one of the main causes of pain during labour was fear of giving birth, and he brought the principles of natural childbirth to the attention of not only the medical world, but to parents as well. He introduced proper education of mothers through antenatal classes and teaching, and also provided emotional support, with the idea of eliminating fear and tension.

His teaching was so fundamental that it is now taken for granted by all centres, and there is no method of childbirth that does not rely on his ideas, which included breathing exercises, breathing control, and complete relaxation. Dr Dick-Read's watchword was preparation – pregnant women need to prepare for birth not only by getting information about childbirth, but also by seeking reassurance and sympathy.

Frederick Leboyer

The Leboyer method of delivery is best understood as an attempt to help people understand what the newborn baby sees, hears, and feels. Leboyer was influenced by the psychiatrists Reich, Rank, and Janov, who shared the belief that problems later in life stem from shock experienced during the process of birth. Leboyer's concern, therefore, is not primarily with the mother, but rather with the baby's experience of delivery.

His book, *Birth Without Violence* (1975), states that in order to minimize the traumatic effects of birth, the birthing room should have soft lighting, and that noise and movement should be kept to a minimum. Leboyer also believes that immediate skin-to-skin contact is essential to calm the baby, and she should be laid on her mother's stomach as soon as she is born. He suggests that the newborn should then be bathed in warm water as this is close to the internal environment of the uterus.

Not all of this fits in with the physiology of what actually occurs at birth. A baby needs the shock of feeling cool air on her skin to make her gasp and fill her lungs with her first breath: placing her in a warm liquid doesn't accomplish this kick-start. Many professionals say that there is no proof that Leboyer's theories work. However, it is only right that every baby be welcomed into the world with reverence, so even if you don't agree with all of Leboyer's theories, it is still interesting to read about his suggestions for a gentler birth.

Dr Michel Odent

As a surgeon, Dr Odent was extremely shocked when he first saw women on their backs with their feet held in stirrups, pushing their babies out against the force of gravity. This traditional delivery position meant that stronger, more painful contractions were needed to push the baby uphill, labour was slower and more exhausting, and patients were more likely to suffer complications.

This led him to devise his own methods of childbirth, broadly based on traditional midwifery, at Pithiviers Hospital in France. Odent believes that, given the opportunity, women in labour return to a primitive biological state where they function at a new level of awareness and follow their basic instincts. He believes that endorphins, the body's natural narcotics, are responsible for this.

Using his methods, Pithiviers has the lowest rate in France for episiotomy, forceps delivery, and Caesarean section, and all interference is kept to a minimum.

Sheila Kitzinger

A very highly respected birth practitioner, Kitzinger believes that birth is a personal experience, and that the labouring mother should be an active "birth-giver", rather than a passive patient.

She believes that maternity services must allow parents to have a real choice, whether it be a totally managed birth, a totally natural birth, or somewhere in between, and that it's essential to respect parents' wishes. She also believes that birth is not an illness, and that professionals must not treat a labouring mother and her partner as patients, but as intelligent adults whose right it is to have the final say in decisions surrounding the birth of their baby.

The Lamaze method

This method of psychological counselling was pioneered in Russia, and then adopted by Dr Lamaze in France.

Over 90 per cent of women in Russia and 70 per cent of French women are now taught variations of the Lamaze method. It has become equally popular in the United States, and still forms the basic teaching of the National Childbirth Trust in the UK.

Lamaze felt that no matter how relaxed a woman was, she would almost certainly experience some pain, and that she would have to cope with it.

Following the reporting of Ivan Pavlov's research into stimulus-response conditioning in dogs, Lamaze saw the value of conditioned learning in helping women cope with the pain of childbirth.

The method has three mainstays. The first is that your fear of labour is reduced or eliminated by information and understanding. Second, you learn how to relax and become aware of your body, and therefore, how to cope with pain. Third, you consciously use rhythmic breathing patterns through each contraction in order to distract your mind from the pain.

Thoughts
on childbirth

Your choices in childbirth

Most of the influential birth philosophers (see pp. 36–37) have been concerned with natural childbirth.

Natural childbirth means normal physiological childbirth. When childbirth becomes associated with varying degrees of fear and therefore varying degrees of tension, it becomes in varying degrees unphysiological or pathological.
Grantley Dick-Read

Doctors and midwives, once they have become aware of the ordeal it is to be born, will meet the young newcomer with more sensitivity, more intelligence, and more respect.
Frederick Leboyer

Everywhere around us, we saw doctors increasing their use of drugs and artificial intervention, while we have kept intervention to an absolute minimum, and considered drugs unnecessary and harmful.
Michel Odent

Childbirth is not primarily a medical process, but a psychosexual experience. It is not surprising that adapting your responses to the stimuli it presents should involve a subtle and delicate working together of mind and body.
Sheila Kitzinger

Over the past few decades, women have been taking greater control of their own health. In many cases, members of the medical profession have responded enthusiastically to the changing desires and needs of women, and the mother's "choices" in childbirth have never been greater, nor her wishes more paramount. Today, most women ask to have their children more naturally, and this option should be available to all of them, whether the birth is at home or in hospital. But women shouldn't ignore the benefits a managed birth can provide, particularly when childbirth doesn't go as smoothly as expected.

Managed or high-tech birth

The modern managed or high-tech birth in hospital came out of a justified concern for the mother and baby, and from increased medical knowledge of the physiological aspects of birth. In a managed birth, labour is actively controlled so that it fits into what is perceived as being normal (this perception can differ, however, depending on the hospital and the obstetrician).

A managed labour is the norm for most hospital births and it is essential for those women who have complications during pregnancy, labour, or birth – for example, if you have high blood pressure or an anticipated breech birth. In these situations, you'll have more antenatal check-ups in hospital, which can mean that you are seen by different doctors and midwives at each visit.

In this setting, you are most likely to experience medical intervention involving some of the most modern procedures in obstetrics. With this kind of labour, epidural anaesthesia is literally on tap and electronic fetal monitoring is standard. Your attendants will notice even very small changes in your baby's condition and may be pressured to act on such changes. Consequently, with this type of birth, there are more inductions and Caesareans, and more frequent use of forceps and vacuum devices.

Although these practices are beneficial to a percentage of births where intervention is necessary, the routine use of them often cannot be justified by hard evidence, so women who want to have complete control over their deliveries may feel very strongly about their use. However, some women feel that a hospital setting makes childbirth the event they expect it to be, and they would feel cheated, nervous, or even second-class if they didn't have an obstetrician in attendance with high-tech equipment close by.

Natural childbirth

It seems a paradox that you have to request a natural birth, but even today you may find that childbirth is still dominated by obstetricians and a few old-fashioned midwives. However, if you make your preferences known early, you can plan to have as natural a birth as possible.

It is reasonable for women to want to have a natural birth in which there is no fear because the whole process of delivery and birth is familiar, where there is no unnecessary medical intervention, where there is a calm, homely atmosphere, and where mothers are allowed to do anything they desire – to take up whatever position is most comfortable and not be under pressure to take pain-relieving drugs. Female bodies are well designed for giving birth: all the soft tissues of the birth passage can open up so that the baby is gently squeezed out. But breathing and relaxation techniques can make birth even easier to manage, and a number of natural childbirth philosophies advocate these techniques.

Although there are individual differences, all birth philosophies share one common aim – to allow women to give birth in the way they want. They emphasize the need for intense concentration on breathing patterns and the learned ability to relax the body at will. The best way to experience a totally natural birth is in a dedicated centre or at home.

Home birth

In many countries, healthy women can opt for a home delivery if their pregnancy has been straightforward. In the UK, it is less easy. When considering a home birth, most doctors would like you to have had one normal child by a normal delivery before agreeing to a home birth for a second baby. Arranging a home birth can be difficult (see column, right), and you must be very sure that it is the best option for you. Keep an open mind about transferring to a hospital if things do not progress well during labour.

Are home births safe?

A planned home birth can be one of the safest ways you can give birth.

A recent British report has concluded that although 94 per cent of all births take place in hospitals, they are no safer, and may be less safe, than home births.

In Australia, a study of 3,400 home births found that there was a lower perinatal mortality rate and less need for Caesareans, forceps, and suturing for an episiotomy or a tear than in hospital deliveries. The mothers were not all "low risk": the group included 15 multiple births, breech deliveries, women who had had Caesareans, and women with previous stillbirths. The group as a whole was older than the national average.

Planning a home birth
Arranging a home birth isn't always straightforward, but if it's what you want it's worthwhile to try.

* Visit your doctor and request a home birth.

* If your doctor agrees, arrange antenatal visits.

* If your doctor says no without a solid medical reason, find a midwife through your hospital or the Independent Midwives' Association (see p. 77).

* Arrange antenatal visits as usual with your new carer.

Your home birth

At home, pre-labour will shift imperceptibly into full labour, without changes in location or your attendants.

✳ You will remain in familiar surroundings with no need to travel while in labour.

✳ Once notified, your midwife will come to your house and stay with you throughout.

✳ You will be free to move around and take up any position that feels comfortable.

✳ You will be encouraged to take your own time during labour.

✳ Your membranes will usually be allowed to rupture spontaneously.

✳ You will be encouraged to seek pain relief without drugs, although gas and oxygen, and pethidine are usually available.

✳ Your midwife will try hard to give your vagina time to stretch, so avoiding a tear and the need for an episiotomy.

✳ Your partner and family can be a part of the birth.

✳ You will have your baby with you at all times.

✳ After the birth you will be free to celebrate as you wish.

Home or hospital?

The main difference between a home and a hospital birth is that at home you are the team captain and everyone else is there to support you. You will have the same midwife throughout and you will not be separated from your baby or your partner afterwards. On the other hand, if you are in hospital, emergency medical assistance is immediately available should anything go wrong.

Home birth

During the early stages of labour, you will probably find that it is more comfortable if you move around. Once labour has become established, you or your partner should phone the midwife, if she isn't already on her way, as well as any other people you want to be present.

When the midwife arrives Your midwife will ask about your progress and examine you. She will be with you throughout labour and she will monitor the baby every five minutes with a Sonicaid (see p. 61). Along with your partner, she will encourage you and help you into the most comfortable positions; some pain relief will be available if you need it.

Giving birth As the baby is being born, you will probably find it helpful to squat. Your partner may "catch" the baby before placing him onto your abdomen. The baby's cord will be clamped, and cut once it has stopped pulsating, then he will be quickly checked over, and the midwife will help you deliver the placenta.

A little later, the baby will be given a thorough examination and weighed on a spring scale. You will be cleaned up and if necessary, sutured. Then you can become acquainted with your new family member.

There are certain clear advantages to having your baby at home, such as the security of being in familiar surroundings with all the privacy you require. Your partner can play an integral part in the birth and your other children may also be present. You will avoid routine medical intervention. At home, you won't have to perform according to preconceived medical ideas of what is normal. Disadvantages include the fact that if something does go seriously wrong, you will have to go into hospital.

Hospital birth

Most babies are born in hospital. Although more women are choosing to have babies at home, the majority of them, encouraged by their medical advisers or their own predilections, will give birth in hospital.

What to expect The unfamiliarity of hospital surroundings can add to the drama of the occasion, but you should be given a chance to look around the facility and meet the staff before you are admitted, and with a birth partner to give you support and your own comfort aids, such as music, the experience should be more pleasurable.

These days, most hospitals are more relaxed about making you feel comfortable during labour. Trading your own clothes for a hospital gown can be de-personalizing, so if this bothers you, find out beforehand if you can wear your own nightdress or a T-shirt. If you normally wear contact lenses, tell the hospital because they may prefer you to wear spectacles during the delivery.

After admission When you arrive at the hospital, your doctor or midwife will ask you about the progress of labour, examine your abdomen to confirm the situation, feel the baby's position, and check the baby's heart. You'll be given an internal examination to see how far your cervix has dilated. Fetal monitoring equipment may be set up. It can be awkward to move around once the equipment is attached, so you may have to stay in one place.

Giving birth If you have decided that you would prefer to manage without drugs for as long as possible during labour, the midwives will be happy to help you cope by using other methods. Drug relief, such as epidural anaesthesia, is usually available if it is needed.

If you are in any danger of tearing, an episiotomy (an incision that helps deliver the baby's head) may be performed as the head is crowning. Your baby will be delivered onto your abdomen, and while you take your first look at each other, you will be given an injection into your thigh so that your uterus contracts, thus helping to expel the placenta. Your baby will then be checked over and weighed while you are cleaned up. If you need stitches, you are usually sutured by the midwife at this point, although in some hospitals you may have to wait for a doctor to do this.

Your hospital birth

Your experience of giving birth will vary depending on your choice of hospital and professional attendants (see pp. 22–23), but will probably include the following procedures. If you wish your labour to be different, bring a birth plan (see p. 52) or talk to your doctor or midwife.

* You will probably travel to hospital while you are in labour.

* You will go through brief hospital admission procedures.

* If necessary, your membranes may be ruptured and fetal monitoring equipment set up.

* If labour slows down or stops, you will probably be given syntocinon (see p. 66) in order to stimulate contractions.

* Pain-relieving drugs of different types, including epidural anaesthesia, are usually available.

* Your birth partner will usually be allowed to stay with you during labour and the birth.

* You will probably be attended by shifts of different midwives and doctors, especially if you are in labour into the night.

* You will probably be given an injection to help you deliver the placenta.

* You will be given your baby to hold immediately after the birth and encouraged to start breastfeeding.

ᵞour
considerations

There are many things that you need to think about or investigate when you are selecting the hospital in which to give birth. Here are some questions to ask yourself and your doctor or midwife before you decide:

✳ What sort of birth do I want – active, natural, or managed?

✳ What birth facilities are on offer in my area?

✳ Am I prepared, or able, to travel for antenatal care? Can it be provided by my doctor?

✳ What sort of reputation do the hospitals in my area have?

✳ What are the staff at the different hospitals actually like? What are their views on labour and birth? Do I agree with them?

✳ Do I want a special care baby unit to be available immediately?

✳ How long do I want to be in hospital, and what sort of rooming-in facilities are available?

✳ Do I want to feed my baby whenever and however I want, without pressure?

✳ Do I want my baby with me at night? All night?

✳ What are the visiting hours?

✳ Can my partner (and children) be with me whenever I want?

✳ Can my partner stay with me the first night after the birth?

Selecting a hospital

Information about the hospitals in your area can be acquired from your doctor, antenatal clinic, social worker, and friends and acquaintances. However, the only way to find out what a hospital can offer you, and whether you feel it is right for you, is to visit it and ask questions. Take a list of questions with you and make sure you get satisfactory answers so that you can come to a confident and wholehearted decision.

Which hospital

There are various kinds of hospital, most of which provide maternity care. The most modern facilities are found in larger hospitals, where doctors are always on duty, so if you run into any complications, one will attend to you. In general, doctors at teaching hospitals are usually more experienced in dealing with complicated births.

Smaller community units tend to be more friendly and flexible. There is much less red tape because there are fewer staff and patients; it's easier to meet the people who can help you, and there's no doubt that you will be able to arrange a more personalized childbirth.

Visit the hospital

To help you make your choice, the first thing to do is to visit one or more hospitals with your birth partner. There may be a formal maternity tour, often as part of the hospital's antenatal classes, but if not, ask for a personal tour accompanied by a member of staff who knows the hospital well. If the hospital will not allow you to see the facilities, ask questions. If they're rigid in their approach to visitors, they are likely to be equally rigid in their approach to maternity care.

The hospital's procedures

Once you have decided, it is a good idea to visit the hospital of your choice again so that you can meet the staff who will be looking after you and become familiar with the delivery room and other facilities. If, after discussion with the staff, you find that your hospital is not able to live up to your expectations, remember that a hospital is there to serve you, and you do have the right to refuse certain procedures. If the hospital is unwilling to listen to your point of view, you can arrange for a transfer to a different one, or opt for another type of care, such as that provided by a family-oriented hospital (see below). If, however, your midwife is part of one of the team midwife schemes (see p. 23), she will come into the hospital with you and deliver your baby there; the hospital staff are only rarely involved. If all goes well, you will be discharged within a few hours and need have little to do with the hospital's procedures.

Natural birthing units

Quite a few hospitals now have birthing units that are less clinical and more like your own home, with comfortable chairs, piles of cushions on which you can arrange yourself, low lighting, soft music, and even drinks and snacks in case you are thirsty or hungry. Family-oriented maternity care is a philosophy aimed at nurturing the family unit during labour and delivery, and after birth.

The whole aim of a birthing unit is to help the mother relax, overcome fears, and relieve tension. A normal routine prior to birth makes for a normal delivery, and once you're in a birthing unit you will not be moved unless an emergency occurs that requires immediate attention. This method prevents uncomfortable breaks with a jarring change of movement, mood, and surroundings. It's not necessary to lie down to have your baby or be surrounded by rather intimidating technological paraphernalia. In a birthing unit you can take up whatever position you feel comfortable in to give birth to your baby. Many units encourage the use of water to help relieve pain, and offer baths or bathing pools.

For many women, a birthing unit provides the ideal compromise between home and hospital births as it provides surroundings and facilities similar to those at home, but emergency expertise and equipment are available if the need arises.

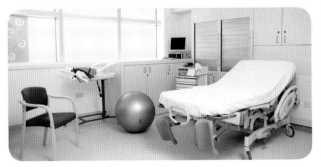

Your birthing room Take your time choosing your hospital, as this is where you are going to give birth to your baby and be taken care of. Make sure you are absolutely convinced about the staff and facilities before you decide.

What to ask the hospital

Once you have chosen a hospital, find out as much as you can by asking questions.

* Will I be able to wear my own clothes and personal effects (rings, contact lenses, glasses)?

* Can my partner or friend stay with me throughout?

* Will I be able to move around freely during labour and give birth in any position I choose?

* Will I be able to have the same carers throughout labour?

* Can I bring in my own midwife to attend to me throughout labour?

* Does the hospital have a natural birthing unit? Are beanbags, stools, and birthing chairs provided?

* Does the hospital offer birthing pools? If not, will I be able to use a hired one?

* What is the hospital policy on pain relief, routine electronic monitoring, and induction?

* What kind of pain relief is used? Is it available at all times?

* Will I be able to eat and drink if I want to?

* What is the hospital policy on procedures such as episiotomies, Caesareans, and the expulsion of the placenta?

* What is the hospital policy on the separation of parents and child in the first hour after birth or later?

Preparing for a home birth

When you opt for a home birth, your midwife will give you detailed advice on the preparations you need to make. Think about what you will need for a home birth about four weeks in advance of your due date, so that you do not have to rush around getting everything organized at the last minute, and you are at least partly prepared if your baby comes early.

Your birthing room

Your bedroom, or whichever room you intend to give birth in, should be arranged so that it is quiet, warm, convenient, and comfortable for you. Put the bed at right angles to the wall, with plenty of space on each side so that the midwife has easy access.

Facilities for your midwife Ideally, you should provide your midwife with a small side table or a tea trolley next to the bed, on which she can put her instruments and other equipment, although a couple of tea trays will do just as well. She will also need a bright, adjustable reading lamp so that she can direct light on to your perineum. A torch (with spare batteries and bulb) would be useful to have at hand in case of a power cut. You should also make sure that you stock up on snacks and drinks in the few days before you are due. Remember that you will need to provide food for your midwife and your birth attendant, too.

Getting the room ready Whether you deliver your baby on to the floor or the bed, the area below and immediately around you will need to be protected during the birth. Have some old, clean sheets, towels, or plastic sheeting ready so that they can be put down when the time comes. Plastic sheeting is available from your local builders' merchant, although an old shower curtain or plastic tablecloth would be fine to use instead.

When labour has begun

You can be sure labour has begun when your contractions are coming every 15 minutes or less, are about one minute long, and don't die away when you move around. This is the time

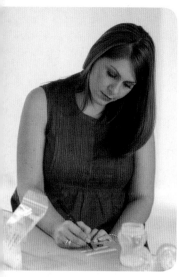

Advance preparation To avoid last-minute panic, make a list of everything you will need well in advance.

to telephone your midwife. It is common for first labours to take a while to get going, so although your midwife will want to know that things have started happening, she is likely to advise you to try and relax and get some rest until you are in full labour, because it is important to conserve your energy. All independent midwives can be contacted by mobile phone, so it is easy to keep in touch. Contact your birth partner if he or she is not already with you. You also need to make arrangements for someone to look after any other children you may have.

Final preparations Make sure everything you and the midwife will need for the birth and immediately afterwards is prepared and ready at hand – including bowls for washing, a bedpan (or a clean bucket), clean towels, and large plastic bags for the soiled dressings. Then put out a clean nightdress or a large T-shirt for yourself, air the baby's clothes, and prepare the baby's cot. Once your midwife and birth attendant have arrived, it is a good idea to turn off your mobile and take the telephone off the hook.

Your midwife's equipment The delivery equipment she brings will include a sphygmomanometer to take blood pressure, Sonicaid to listen to the baby's heart, Entonox (gas and oxygen) cylinder, urine-testing sticks, local anaesthetic and syringes, scissors, suture material, mucus extractor, resuscitation equipment, intravenous equipment (in case of bleeding), and syntometrine. If you wish to have pain-relieving drugs, such as pethidine, she will arrange for a prescription to collect it in advance.

Going to hospital unexpectedly With the help of a skilled midwife or doctor, a home birth is completely safe for both you and your baby. But, as is also the case with hospital births, there can be complications, and if there's a serious problem you might have to go into hospital instead of having your baby at home. If that should happen, your midwife or doctor will go with you.

It can be bitterly disappointing if you can't give birth at home after all your plans, but if you and your partner consider this possibility and talk about it in advance, it'll be easier to cope with if you do have to transfer to hospital. It's better to tell yourself that you're going to start your labour at home and see how it goes before deciding where your baby will actually be born.

When not to have a home birth

Normally, it is as safe to give birth at home as it is in a hospital, but in certain circumstances a hospital birth is your only option.

There are a number of factors that can make a hospital birth necessary. Some, such as diabetes, will mean that you have to plan on a hospital delivery; others, which occur suddenly, such as placental abruption, will mean that you have to abandon your plans for a home birth and go immediately to hospital. The factors that rule out a home birth include:

* When you have had complications in any of your previous pregnancies.

* When your pelvis is too small for your baby's head to pass through.

* When your baby is presenting in the breech position.

* When you have a medical problem that puts you, your baby, or both of you at risk, such as high blood pressure, anaemia, diabetes, excess amniotic fluid, active herpes, placenta praevia, placental abruption, or pre-eclampsia.

* When you have a multiple pregnancy.

* When your baby is premature.

* When your pregnancy goes well beyond your estimated delivery date.

Childbirth teachers

You'll probably choose a childbirth teacher or class fairly early in your pregnancy; make plans to start classes in your seventh month or earlier. In most cases, you will have to book a place.

Both the quality and approach of classes can vary – some are tightly structured, with little question-and-answer time, others allow plenty of time to practise techniques. Some depend mainly on lectures, others on class participation. The teacher is very often the determining factor so, if you can, check with other couples you know who have attended classes before you make your final choice.

Try to select a teacher whose philosophy of birth fits in with the type of birth you'd like to have. Conflicts and confusion can arise if what you learn in class does not accord with your later experience in hospital or at home.

Find out how many couples are taught in each class. Half a dozen couples is ideal, because you will receive plenty of attention from the teacher while getting to know your fellow participants.

Most childbirth teachers will be very happy to talk to you about their approach – even if you are not yet attending childbirth classes.

Childbirth classes

As an enthusiastic proponent of prepared childbirth, I believe that everyone can benefit from childbirth or parentcraft classes. These classes can be tremendously enjoyable. The camaraderie is wonderful and you may find that the other members of the group act as a substitute for your extended family as you exchange experiences; certainly they will make you feel less alone and isolated. It's a great benefit to be able to share one's thoughts and feelings with people who are in the same position and it helps to relieve tension and anxiety. Strong personal bonds are often formed with others in these classes that can be the basis of lasting friendships. It's important for your partner to go with you to these classes; most prospective fathers find them very useful.

Topics covered

Childbirth or parentcraft classes are particularly useful for first-time parents because they're designed to give you information that will make you both feel more confident. They work in three ways.

First, they cover the processes of pregnancy and birth, including female anatomy and physiology, and the changes that occur throughout pregnancy. This is done so that you have a clearer understanding of what is involved and why things are happening. Your teacher will also talk to you about the sort of medical procedures that you can expect and why these will be done.

Second, the classes provide practical instruction in relaxation, breathing, and exercising techniques (see pp. 48–49) that can help you to control your labour and reduce pain, and will also give you the confidence that only comes with being familiar with what's happening. Bear in mind that bodies, not brains, give birth, so anything that helps you tune into your body is going to be useful. Your partner should also learn how to give you a massage to help relieve pain.

Third, your teacher will talk you through the stages of labour and birth, and aspects of postnatal recovery. You will be advised on breastfeeding, making up formula, and bottlefeeding. Both you and your partner can practise changing nappies and bathing and dressing a baby. This will help you cope with the practicalities of babycare.

Exercise classes

Doing exercises that strengthen the muscles used in childbirth often results in an easier delivery (see p. 48). Many hospitals offer antenatal classes that incorporate exercise and relaxation techniques, and there are independent organizations as well – some are even meant for specific types of birth. If you tell your instructor that you would like to have your baby in a standing or squatting position, for example, you will be given suitable exercises to help strengthen the muscles in your back, hips, and legs.

Techniques for easier childbirth

Studies have shown that taking childbirth classes shortens the length of labour. In one study, the average duration of labour for a group of women who had taken classes was 13.56 hours, compared with the average labour of 18.33 hours in the control group, which had no training. This is probably because knowing how to deal with pain produces a more relaxed labour. Strategies for dealing with pain include the following:

Cognitive control You dissociate your mind from the pain by visualizing a pleasant scenario in which to experience the pain; for example, when you feel pain you imagine your baby moving further down the birth canal, closer to emerging. In this way, you will be concentrating on the non-painful part of the sensation.

Systematic relaxation In order to increase your tolerance of pain, you are taught exercises to relax the various muscles of the body (see p. 49). In this way, you will be able to isolate pain from the contracting uterus rather than allowing it to pervade the rest of your body.

Hawthorne rehearsal You receive enhanced attention from a birth assistant. Psychological research has shown that the more attention you are given, the less pain you feel.

Hypnobirthing One fairly new approach that you may like to consider is hypnobirthing, where you'll be prepared for birth by a trained hypnotherapist during five or so 30-minute visits throughout your pregnancy. Careful research has shown that hypnosis can help you deal with pain, avoid complications, and reduce postnatal depression.

The dad's role

In an antenatal class, you may be able to show your partner for the first time just how central a role he is going to play.

Classes will make a supportive man a more effective birth partner by familiarizing him with the processes of labour and delivery.

Some courses have father-only sessions where the men can talk freely about any problems or anxieties they have about the forthcoming event. A worried man can find security and support in the company of other fathers-to-be.

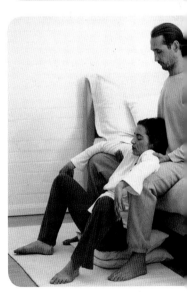

Team effort Childbirth classes give a couple a unique opportunity to work as a team towards a common goal – the birth of their baby – and this often results in a special closeness.

Your pelvic floor

The pelvic floor muscles form a funnel that supports the uterus, bowel, and bladder, and serves to close the entrances to the vagina, rectum, and urethra.

During pregnancy, an increase in progesterone causes the muscles to soften and relax. To counter this there is an exercise you can do to keep the pelvic floor well toned and also prevent later problems.

Pull up and tense the muscles around your vagina and anus, as if you were stopping the flow of urine. Hold as long as you can without straining. Relax. Repeat 25 times a day.

You should restart this exercise as soon as you can after delivery to minimize the risk of prolapse. Early exercise will tone up the vagina for sexual intercourse, too. Make this part of your daily routine.

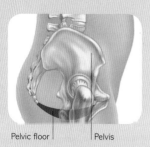

Pelvic floor   Pelvis

Preparation for labour

As you approach your delivery date, your childbirth classes will help you prepare for labour. You can also get yourself ready by practising pelvic floor exercises and breathing techniques, and learning how to relax.

Pelvic floor exercises

During pregnancy and delivery, your pelvic floor (see column, left) can be stretched by the weight of the baby, which may cause discomfort and problems after the birth. You should perform pelvic floor exercises all through pregnancy and immediately after birth to keep the muscles of your pelvic floor firm and toned.

Breathing techniques

It's worth mastering breathing techniques because they are extremely useful during labour. In the first place, they give you a wonderful feeling of control over your body. But also, miraculously almost, breathing can increase your ability to cope with pain.

Any woman who wants to at least try natural childbirth can learn breathing exercises that may help her to get through labour without resorting to painkillers or anaesthetics. In addition, deep breathing will calm you, prevent you from becoming fearful, and therefore help to conserve energy that you will need for bearing down. Each of the different levels of breathing is useful at a different point during labour. Make sure that your birth partner is familiar with them, too, so that he can support and encourage you during labour.

Deep breathing The point of this kind of breathing is to fill the deepest point of your lungs with air so that your brain and the placenta receive plenty of oxygen. You should feel your ribcage lift upwards and outwards as you inhale. A trick I learned was to take in as much breath as I could and then, at the last moment, breathe in a little more. Then, if you drop your shoulders, the elastic recoil of your lungs will push the air slowly out. Concentrate on exhaling; it will help if your birth partner wraps his arms around your lower back and you let your ribs sink, with a sigh, into his cupped hands. This level of breathing is particularly helpful at the beginning and end of contractions.

Feather-light breathing I use this kind of breathing to prepare myself whenever I have to make a great physical effort. It's really just rapid panting and it can be useful at any time, but particularly during labour, to aerate the lungs very efficiently over a short space of time. In the transition period you need to do this to stop yourself bearing down before full dilation.

Take shallow breaths in and out so that you sound like a dog panting, using only the upper part of the lungs. After about 10–15 seconds of this, the body feels a blast of oxygen rushing into the system. It's also very effective in eliminating carbon dioxide from your system. But its main use in labour is to distract you – while you are panting you can't do much else. It primes you for action, and incidentally, stops you feeling pain as intensely – so it's excellent at the height of a contraction.

To prevent yourself from overbreathing, hold your breath for a count of five every 10–15 breaths. It is during this breath-holding time in stage two of labour that you would push.

Light breathing This kind of breathing uses the upper half of the lungs to the extent that you feel your shoulders and shoulder-blades rising. You concentrate very hard on breathing in through your mouth and throat with your lips apart and take short, sharp breaths. This level of breathing is useful at the height of a painful contraction. To practise, get your birth partner to place his hands on your upper back so that you get the feel of the movement.

Why relaxation helps

The benefits of learning relaxation techniques are several: they help you to conserve energy during pregnancy by resting instantly whenever you are tired during the day and evening. Even a few minutes of relaxation are refreshing and allow you to make the most of spare moments to replenish your energy. It is also useful during labour to be able to relax your body at will because this will help reduce tension and enhance your ability to tolerate pain.

Mental relaxation is achieved through the skill of physical relaxation. First, clear your mind – my trick is to think of black velvet – and concentrate on calming your breathing. Cut down your rate of breathing by half. If any troublesome thoughts recur, stop them with a mental "no". Then think of the most tranquil scene you can imagine and keep it in your mind's eye. Breathe deeply and slowly the entire time.

Relaxing your body

The benefit of learning to relax the muscles of your body in sequence is that you can isolate yourself from the uterus in labour, so that it alone is contracting, while none of your other muscles is tense.

The best way to isolate a group of muscles is to tense them, feel the tension, then let go. Start by practising twice a day for 15–20 minutes in a comfortable position, sitting or lying with your eyes closed. Work on the muscles in your forehead first. Tense them and then let them relax. Work down your body in sequence – eyes, cheeks, jaw, chin, neck, shoulders, arms, hands – until your whole body feels heavy. A good sign that you are properly relaxed is that you no longer feel whatever you're sitting or lying on is pushing back into your body.

Fit for pregnancy

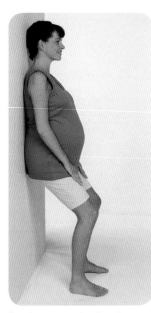

By performing exercises, you will relieve the strain caused by your extra weight and strengthen important muscles. Practise these daily if possible, building repetitions gradually. Don't get overheated while exercising. Remember to drink plenty of water. Stop immediately if anything hurts, or if you feel sick, dizzy, or breathless.

Leg stretches

During pregnancy, your legs have to carry a lot of extra weight, so it's important to stretch and strengthen the muscles. These exercises will also improve the circulation in your legs.

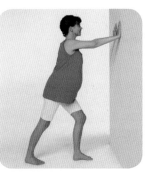

Exercise to strengthen legs Rest against a wall with your feet apart. Slowly bend your legs until you feel some pull on the thigh muscles but before you feel uncomfortable. Stay in this position for a count of 20, then stand up.

Stretching calf muscles Facing a wall, bend your elbows and lean against the wall, with your weight on your hands. Place one foot behind the other, making sure that both feet point at the wall. As you bend one knee, stretch the rear calf muscle. Hold, then release, and repeat with the other leg.

Feet and ankles

Pregnancy hormones relax the walls of the veins, which slows the blood to the heart and can cause varicose veins, and swollen ankles and legs. Do these exercises regularly to stimulate the circulation.

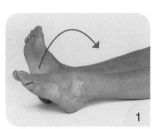

1

1 Foot exercises Flex one foot up and down from the ankle, but do not point the toes (or you may get a cramp). Repeat with the other foot. Do this 10 to 20 times per foot at least twice a day.

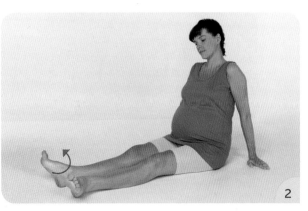

2

2 Circle the feet Gently circle your feet 10 times one way, and again the other way. Remember to keep your toes relaxed.

Pelvic tilt

Do pelvic tilt exercises to strengthen your lower back and abdominal muscles, so preventing bad posture and backache.

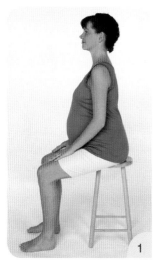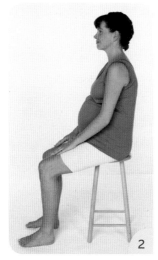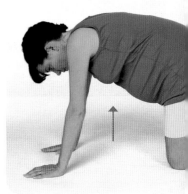

On all fours Breathe in, then exhale and lift your back and pull in your stomach, clenching your buttock muscles. Hold, then release and return your back to a level position, holding your stomach muscles firm. Repeat this several times.

1 **Upright position** With your feet resting flat on the floor, sit on a sturdy stool or chair. Rock your pelvis forward.

2 **Pulling in your stomach** Taking care of your back, pull in your stomach muscles and rock back on your hips. Release. Repeat this several times.

Hips and trunk

Your mobility can be increased by twisting and circling exercises; these loosen the trunk area. You may also find that the hip circling movement (see below) is especially helpful during the first stage of labour to relieve backache.

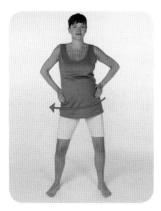

Circling your hips Place your feet apart and have your knees slightly bent, with hands on hips. Slowly circle your hips around in one direction five to 10 times, then repeat in the other direction.

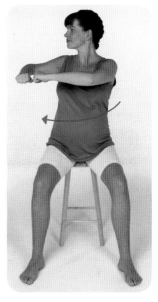

Twisting Sit with your feet flat on the floor and your knees apart. Raise your arms to chest level and twist the upper body to one side as far as you can, then twist to the other. Repeat several times.

Covering your alternatives

Although you will make your plan according to the kind of birth you would like to have, it is a good idea to have another one on stand-by.

This alternative plan can set out the procedures that you would prefer to be followed should complications arise. On rare occasions, labour may become unexpectedly prolonged or difficult, or the baby may need special attention. By considering all the possibilities, you will help your birth attendants to take care of any situation as you would wish.

Your birth plan

Making a plan for your baby's birth will help to ensure that you are actively involved in the way he is born. By carefully considering all your ideas and preferences, and by discussing them with your partner and birth attendants, you will be able to establish a bond of trust and create a happier and more comfortable labour.

A consensus plan

Think about the issues that are important to you and then find out whether what you want is feasible (see pp. 43 and 54). There is no point in making a plan that cannot be used once you are in labour. Discuss your ideas with your GP early in your pregnancy so that he or she can refer you to the consultant obstetrician most likely to accord with your wishes. You should make specific enquiries about the routines followed where you intend to give birth, as some hospitals may not be able to meet your requirements. Also, discuss your ideas with your midwife, antenatal teacher, and other members of your antenatal team as they will be able to advise you about the kinds of experience mothers have had in local hospitals and with particular doctors.

Hospital response Your hospital team may be pleased to see how well you have prepared yourself for the labour and encourage your full participation. Some mothers experience negativity from hospital staff on the grounds that a birth plan interferes with their standard practices. Don't be intimidated – just remember that your baby and the way in which you give birth are your responsibility.

Working together Co-operation is an important feature of the birth plan. By working it out in detail with everyone concerned, you should be able to alleviate any anxieties and feel more in control of your baby's birth. Make sure, too, that the staff know of any alternative plan (see column, left).
Try to maintain a friendly relationship with your professional attendants so that they try to follow your wishes. Give a copy of the plan to your midwife or the hospital team; a copy should also be placed with your hospital records. This is important in case you are attended in labour by someone who doesn't know your wishes.

Presenting your birth plan These two examples of a birth plan outline the different choices of birth – there are many variations. The plan may be laid out as a letter or a simple list. It can be typed or handwritten. Remember to add your name and address and/or hospital number if you have one. Make a note in your birth plan of any special needs, such as diet, which may be applicable during your time in hospital.

Thank you for all the information that you have provided in the antenatal classes and at the childbirth classes. I have thought carefully about how I would like my labour and delivery to be.

My partner, John, will be my companion during labour. He has attended childbirth classes with me.

I understand that electronic fetal monitoring is routinely used and I am happy for this to be done.

If everything goes well and I do not need pain relief, I would prefer to be able to walk around and give birth using a birthing stool, which I will provide myself.

If I need pain relief I would prefer an epidural, with as low an epidural dose as possible so that I still have feeling in my legs and am aware of contractions. I would prefer for it to wear off for the second stage, as I would like to push out the baby myself.

If I have to have a Caesarean section I would like my partner to be with me throughout the operation.

I intend to breastfeed on demand and want the baby to sleep next to me if possible.

Rosita

I am looking forward to coming into Central Hospital. I would like to record a few points about the birth as the midwives have suggested. They are:

Support person — I will be accompanied by my sister, Sarah.

Monitoring — I would prefer to be monitored by a Sonicaid.

Positions — I will probably want to deliver the baby in a semi-upright position, as this is how I had my other two babies.

Pain relief — It is likely that I will need gas and air, as I did last time.

Episiotomy — I would prefer not to be cut if it can be avoided. I would welcome help in order to help prevent it.

Jenna Gatto

Birth plan questions

Before it's possible to express preferences about the way you and your partner would like your birth to be conducted, it is better to be familiar with the routine of the labour ward you have chosen. You will, of course, visit the hospital and talk to the staff about your preferences. It may be difficult to know where to start, so I suggest you draw up a list of questions for your carers before you go. Then write out your plan, working through labour systematically:

✳ How many birth partners am I allowed?
✳ When will labour be induced after the due date?
✳ Can I walk around, eat, and drink during labour?
✳ Will I always be attended by a midwife I know?
✳ If there is a change of staff, will my new midwife be told of my birth plan?
✳ Does a doctor have to be present?
✳ Can my partner and I decide when and what kind of pain relief will be administered?
✳ Does the hospital have epidural anaesthesia, if I want it, available round the clock?
✳ Are there TENS machines (which use electric current to ease the pain) available for hire?
✳ Is a water birth possible?
✳ Can I stand or squat to deliver my baby?
✳ Can I be given enough time to deliver the head so that I don't need an episiotomy?
✳ Can I see my baby's head being delivered?
✳ Can I deliver the rest of my baby myself?
✳ If I have a Caesarean section, can my birth partners come with me to the operating room?
✳ Can we be left alone with the baby after she is born?
✳ Will my placenta be delivered naturally or with an injection of syntometrine?
✳ Who stitches an uncomplicated episiotomy – the midwife, or a doctor?
✳ When can I go home?

When do I write it?

Although you will probably think about the issues involved from early on in your pregnancy, you don't need to finalize your plans until the eighth month.

Chapter 4

Special procedures

Check-ups will be carried out throughout your pregnancy, and if a problem is suspected, **additional tests** will help your doctor to rule out or confirm whether you or your baby need special treatment.

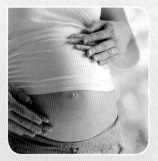
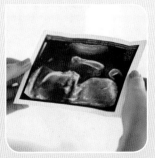
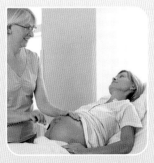

Special tests

If your doctor suspects that there is a problem that cannot be detected by routine tests, or if you have a family history of a particular disorder, you will be asked to undergo further, more specific tests. Apart from enabling doctors to check for various complications, they can perform two useful services for you and your partner: they can be reassuring in giving you and your baby a clean bill of health, and they may provide you with information that may cause you to question whether your pregnancy should proceed. Before making any decision, please have full discussions with your doctor about the tests and results and take advantage of the counsellors who are there to help you.

Chorionic villus sampling (CVS)

The chorionic villi are finger-like outgrowths of the chorion, which form the baby's side of the placenta; they are genetically identical to the fetus. As they develop earlier than the amniotic fluid, examining a sample of chorionic villi will provide information about your baby's genes and chromosomes some weeks before amniocentesis is possible.

Why is it done? The most important group of mothers needing CVS are those at risk of having a Down's syndrome baby. An abnormality of haemoglobin, such as sickle-cell

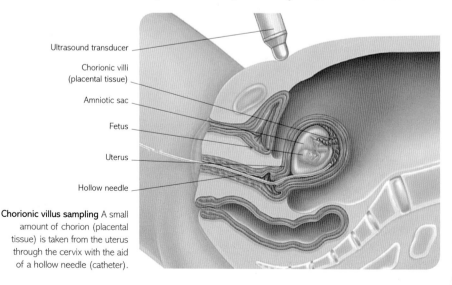

Ultrasound transducer

Chorionic villi (placental tissue)

Amniotic sac

Fetus

Uterus

Hollow needle

Chorionic villus sampling A small amount of chorion (placental tissue) is taken from the uterus through the cervix with the aid of a hollow needle (catheter).

disease or thalassaemia, can also be diagnosed with CVS. Hereditary metabolic disorders are fortunately rare, but if a family is affected, the frequency may be as high as one in four. The basic defect is an enzyme deficiency, and direct enzyme analysis of the chorionic tissue will provide the diagnosis within two days. Single gene disorders, such as cystic fibrosis, haemophilia, Huntington's chorea, and muscular dystrophy, can be detected by microscopic analysis of chorionic villi.

How is it done? CVS is carried out under ultrasound control, usually between 10 and 12 weeks, before the amniotic sac completely fills the uterine cavity. For this procedure, one of two routes is employed: the trans-cervical route or the trans-abdominal route.

For the trans-cervical route (see diagram, p. 56), a plastic or metal hollow needle (catheter) is introduced through the cervical canal into the outside edge of the placenta. A small amount of chorionic villi tissue is removed. The trans-abdominal procedure is similar to that of amniocentesis, but the sample is taken from the placental tissue instead of the amniotic fluid.

The risk of miscarriage following CVS is about two per cent higher than the spontaneous miscarriage rate. The advantage of CVS is that it can be performed earlier than amniocentesis.

Amniocentesis

Amniotic fluid contains cells from the baby's skin and other organs, which provide clues to his condition. Amniocentesis is the simple procedure that withdraws this fluid from the uterus.

Why is it done? You may be offered an amniocentesis if you have a previous baby with Down's syndrome, if your blood tests have revealed a very low level of alpha-fetoprotein (see p. 31), or if there is a thickened nuchal pad on the ultrasound scan. In addition, amniocentesis can reveal other important information if there is already cause for concern. The test shows:

* The sex of the baby: fetal skin cells accumulate in the amniotic fluid. Under the microscope, these cells reveal the baby's sex. In genetically-linked disorders, such as haemophilia, a male child has a 50 per cent chance of being affected. Knowing the baby is male may lead you to decide to terminate the pregnancy, for example, in the

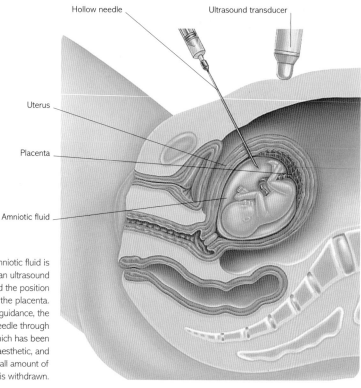

Hollow needle

Ultrasound transducer

Uterus

Placenta

Amniotic fluid

Amniocentesis Amniotic fluid is extracted only after an ultrasound scan has determined the position of the fetus and the placenta. Using ultrasound for guidance, the doctor passes a needle through the abdominal wall, which has been numbed with local anaesthetic, and into the uterus. A small amount of amniotic fluid is withdrawn.

case of haemophilia and some forms of muscular dystrophy.
✳ The chemical composition of the fluid: this can reveal metabolic disorders caused by missing or defective enzymes.
✳ The bilirubin content of the fluid: this helps determine whether a Rhesus-positive baby needs an intrauterine blood transfusion because of Rhesus incompatibility (see p. 62).
✳ The chromosome count: determined by examining discarded cells. Deviation from the normal chromosomal structure may mean that the baby will be handicapped in some way. Conditions include Down's syndrome, Edward's syndrome, and Patau's syndrome, all caused by the baby having an extra chromosome.

How is it done? Amniocentesis is usually performed between 14 and 20 weeks, although it can be done a little earlier. A hollow needle is inserted into the amniotic sac through the front of the abdominal wall and a small amount of fluid is withdrawn. This is then spun in a centrifuge to separate the cells shed by the baby from the rest of the liquid. The cells are cultured for about two to five weeks, and therefore the results take some time. Slightly less accurate results can, however, be available in a few days. The risk of the procedure inducing a miscarriage is about one in 100.

Umbilical vein sampling (cordocentesis)

This procedure is carried out at about 20 weeks or later, often following the ultrasound scan at this time. It is used to examine the constituents of the baby's blood and, in the case of fetal anaemia, to determine whether an intrauterine blood transfusion is necessary. It is also vital in four other situations:

Detecting infection Rubella (German measles), toxoplasmosis, and the herpes virus may be detected by performing a specific radio analysis of certain proteins that are present in the blood of the fetus.

Rhesus iso-immunization In cases of Rhesus incompatibility (see p. 62), the direct assessment of fetal haemoglobin is the best way to determine whether the baby is coping or becoming anaemic, and whether an intrauterine blood transfusion (also done through the umbilical vein) needs to be carried out.

Chromosome count Analysis of certain white blood cells (fetal lymphocytes) will detect chromosomal abnormalities that are associated with Down's syndrome and other conditions. The results take a few days to come through.

Suspected growth restriction If the fetus is considered to be growth-restricted, cordocentesis may be used to measure the acidity or alkalinity of the blood, the amount of oxygen and carbon dioxide, and the amount of bicarbonate in the blood. In addition, plasma levels of glucose can be estimated.

How is it done? Under ultrasonic control, a hollow needle is passed through the front wall of the abdomen and uterus into a blood vessel in the umbilical cord, about 1 centimetre (½ inch) from where it emerges from the placenta. A small quantity of blood can then be removed for testing. Some results can be available immediately, others may take a week or more. The risk to the fetus appears to be about one to two per cent.

Other tests for chromosomal defects

Triple test This is a screening blood test (see p. 30) that was originally developed at St Bartholomew's Hospital in London. A maternal blood sample is taken at 16 weeks to measure the levels of three substances: oestriol, alpha-fetoprotein, and human chorionic gonadotrophin (hCG). The results can be assessed, along with your age, to predict the chance of your baby suffering from Down's syndrome. If it seems high, amniocentesis (see p. 57) is then offered. All women in the UK are now offered this.

Ultrasound scanning Down's syndrome and other chromosomal defects can be suggested by an ultrasound scan of the fetus called a nuchal scan (see p. 34). This investigates the size and shape of the pad at the back of the fetus' neck and can suggest that a defect may be present. If so, amniocentesis or CVS will be offered.

The effect of your age

Your age is an important factor in how your baby develops, but it's just one of several factors that can affect the outcome of your pregnancy; your lifestyle and nutrition are much more important. However, the older you are when you become pregnant, the more likely you are to require special attention. You'll be asked questions to identify whether you have any problems, and appropriate tests will be offered to rule out certain disorders (see below).

Down's syndrome Maternal age does seem to be an important factor in what causes Down's syndrome, although parents of any age can have a baby with this condition.

Mother's age and Down's syndrome The chart shows that the risk of having a Down's syndrome baby rises rapidly after 35 years of age.

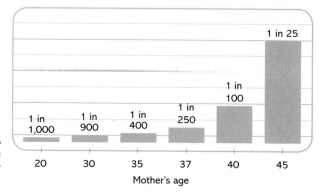

As you can see from the graph (left), the risk of having a baby with Down's syndrome rises with advancing maternal age, but isn't really significant until after 35 years of age. However, as a Down's baby is born every 2,000 births, and as most babies are born to women under 35 who until recently did not undergo screening for Down's syndrome, there are more Down's babies born in the pre-35 age group than in the post-35 age group.

Fetal heart monitoring

This is an efficient method of monitoring the wellbeing of the fetus during pregnancy. A healthy fetus that is receiving an adequate supply of oxygen and nutrients will generally be more active than a malnourished, oxygen-starved fetus, and the heart rate will respond to stress more effectively.

Doctors and midwives use a hand-held monitor called a Sonicaid to check the presence and rate of the heartbeat at every antenatal visit from week 20 onwards. This is a small portable instrument, which uses ultrasound, that is placed on your abdomen. The Sonicaid also magnifies the sound so that you can listen to it.

The baby's heartbeat is much faster than your own (over 120 beats per minute compared with your 75 beats per minute), and sounds just like a tiny galloping horse. When a healthy, active fetus moves, the heart rate accelerates by 15 beats per minute for 15 seconds. If your baby is distressed for any reason, the heart rate drops. Fetal heart monitoring is also useful during labour to detect signs of distress in the baby.

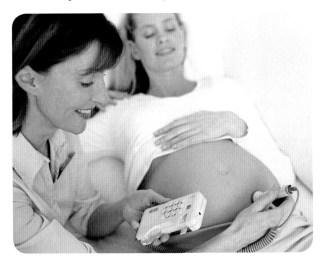

Doppler scan device This special form of ultrasound scan records the movement of red blood cells through blood vessels in the fetus and placenta. It can be used to monitor the heartbeat of the fetus in the womb.

Rhesus incompatibility

Anti-∅ injections

To prevent destructive antibodies from forming and attacking any subsequent babies, pregnant women who are Rhesus-negative need an anti-D injection:

✳ After delivery

✳ After a miscarriage or a termination

✳ After chorionic villus sampling (CVS)

✳ After an amniocentesis or cordocentesis, especially if there is blood on the needle after it has been withdrawn from the uterus

✳ If there is a bleed from the placenta

✳ Routinely at 28 weeks of pregnancy.

About 85 per cent of the population has a substance called the Rhesus factor on their red blood cells. These people are known as Rhesus positive. The remaining 15 per cent, whose blood cells lack the Rhesus factor, are Rhesus negative. Rhesus positivity is always dominant; negativity will exist when only negative genes are inherited. Being Rhesus negative does not affect you unless you are pregnant or need a blood transfusion.

An incompatible mother and baby

In pregnancies where the mother has Rhesus-negative blood and the baby is Rhesus positive (an incompatible pregnancy), the first pregnancy usually goes without a hitch, as the mother's immune system is unlikely to come into contact with the baby's until labour. However, when fetal blood cells mix with maternal cells, for example, during delivery, the mother's blood becomes sensitized.

When the Rh factor from the baby's blood enters the mother's bloodstream, it acts as an antigen and stimulates the production of anti-Rhesus-positive antibodies. These may attack and destroy the blood cells of her next Rhesus-positive (incompatible) baby. This causes haemolytic disease of the newborn, and the infants are affected with blood conditions ranging from mild jaundice to serious, possibly fatal, anaemia. Fetuses that develop the disease can often be saved by an intrauterine blood transfusion.

Not all Rh-negative women with Rh-positive babies become sensitized, but there is no way of predicting which women will. All of these women, therefore, are carefully monitored and given preventative injections in certain situations and after delivery (see column, left).

Careful monitoring

The mother's blood will be monitored throughout her pregnancy. She will have blood taken at 28 weeks to examine for increasing levels of antibodies. Only if the levels increase beyond a certain point is the developing baby in any danger. The antibodies cross over into the baby and can cause a rise in fetal bilirubin (a by-product of red blood cell destruction), and the baby can suffer from severe anaemia. In the third trimester, a direct test for the presence of bilirubin can be done by a process called cordocentesis (see p. 59). This test allows the doctors to assess the severity of the condition and determine whether blood transfusions are necessary.

If the antibody count remains low, the mother will not require further special care. However, if the count rises moderately, her baby may be induced early to prevent serious consequences. In this case, a home birth is out of the question and she will need to deliver in a hospital. In a few cases the baby will have to have a blood transfusion to replace his own blood cells, which have become damaged during pregnancy.

Within 48 hours of delivery, the mother is injected intramuscularly with anti-D to help prevent the destructive antibodies from forming and attacking her next baby.

Rhesus disease in pregnancy

Rhesus disease only occurs when a woman with Rhesus-negative blood (shown as minus signs in the illustration below) is pregnant with a Rhesus-positive (shown as plus signs) baby. Most Rhesus-negative mothers carry their first babies without problems. If they then develop antibodies to Rhesus-positive blood (shown as triangles in the illustration), any subsequent babies could be at risk.

All women who are Rh negative should be offered an anti-D injection at 28 and 34 weeks of pregnancy and after the delivery of a Rh-positive baby. Some units offer a double dose at 28 weeks only. Studies have yet to confirm which is the most effective.

How the baby is affected

The baby is likely to be fit and healthy, owing to the anti-D injections and the special care given during pregnancy.

* Immediately after birth the baby will have a Coomb's test to reveal the presence of maternal anti-Rhesus-positive antibodies.

* If the baby is affected by Rh incompatibility, his levels of bilirubin will rise very quickly after birth because of the liver's poor ability to process it.

* The high level of bilirubin in his blood and tissues will make him look yellow. This can be treated by placing him under a "bili" light, which converts the bilirubin into a harmless substance.

Key
– Rhesus-negative blood
+ Rhesus-positive blood
▲ Antibodies

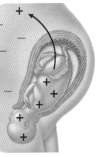

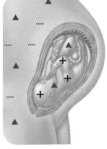

First pregnancy Maternal and fetal blood doesn't usually mix during pregnancy, but during birth the mother may be exposed to her baby's Rh-positive blood.

Mother is sensitized during birth Unless the mother is given an anti-D injection within 48 hours of delivery, she may develop antibodies to Rhesus-positive blood.

Future pregnancy These antibodies will mean that if she becomes pregnant with another Rhesus-positive baby, her antibodies may attack the baby's blood cells.

Your placenta

If your labour does not begin as expected (usually two weeks either side of the EDD), the placenta may then start to become relatively inefficient.

The placenta has substantial reserves, readily adjusts to injury, repairs damages due to ischaemia (lack of oxygen), and does not undergo ageing. There are, however, changes in the character of the villi (small projections around the placenta) during the pregnancy, and by 36 weeks there may be deposits of calcium within the walls of the small blood vessels, and a protein deposit may appear on the surface of many of the villi. These changes can limit the flow of nutrients and waste across the placenta to your baby.

Is my baby overdue?

Only about five per cent of all babies arrive on the date that they are expected. The estimated date of delivery (EDD) is only a statistical average, and studies have shown that as many as 40 per cent of babies are born more than a week after the EDD.

Every pregnancy is different

One of the main difficulties in deciding whether a baby is actually overdue or not is that the precise date of conception in any particular pregnancy is unknown. Even if you have a regular menstrual cycle of 28 days (the standard on which the EDD chart is based), the date of ovulation is only known approximately. Apart from this uncertainty about the date of ovulation, every baby is different and it is therefore unrealistic to expect all babies to mature in precisely the same number of days. Moreover, since labour is initiated by your baby producing certain hormones as he reaches full maturity, it follows that the actual date of delivery can vary fairly widely – even in "textbook" pregnancies.

When labour is delayed

Doctors do become concerned if a pregnancy continues much beyond 10 days after the estimated date of delivery, because post-maturity and possible placental insufficiency pose risks to the health of your baby. The longer the baby continues to grow in the uterus, the larger he is likely to be, which will increase the chances of a difficult labour, and the possibility that the placenta will not be able to continue to support the baby over an extended period.

Post-mature babies

An overdue baby is in danger of being post-mature. A post-mature baby will have lost fat from all over his body, particularly his tummy. Consequently, his skin will look red and wrinkled as if it doesn't fit him, and it may have begun to peel. Very few babies are actually post-mature, but because post-maturity depends not only on the baby, but also on his placenta, it is difficult to predict which babies will be at risk.

What it means The outcome of going well over your due date may include a longer and more difficult labour, because the post-mature baby tends to be bigger and the bones in his skull tend to be harder (which means that his descent through the birth canal is likely to be more traumatic both for him and for you). There is also an increased chance of stillbirth (the risk doubles by the 43rd week and triples by the 44th week). There is a further possibility that a uterus that seems to be slow to start labour may also be relatively inefficient during labour, so that labour is unduly prolonged.

However, doctors are now well aware of the risks of post-mature deliveries and so labour is normally induced 10 days after the estimated delivey date. Post-mature babies are very rare as a result.

Checking that all is well

Babies who have gone past their EDDs are monitored closely, and there are a number of different ways of keeping a check on your baby.

Fetal movement recording One obvious sign that all is well with your baby is if you can detect regular fetal movements. Since all mothers and babies are different, the amount of movement that is normal for each individual pregnancy varies. You are the best judge of whether your unborn baby is acting normally, and you can monitor his activity by making a note of how many kicks you feel in a day.

Electronic fetal monitoring This may be used to check the baby's heartbeat before or during labour. A monitor is strapped around your abdomen. Using ultrasound, it provides a continuous sound or paper recording of the baby's heartbeat. If the heartbeat is satisfactory (particularly during a contraction), doctors usually consider that it is unnecessary to perform other tests, or to induce labour.

Inducing labour

An induced labour is one that is started artificially. Most inductions are elective, which means they are not emergency procedures, but an induced labour may become necessary if your doctor believes you or your baby are at risk, especially if you are well beyond your due date.

If you are in any doubt as to why your doctor is recommending labour be induced, don't hesitate to ask for a detailed explanation – this can involve discussing a range of alternatives to induction.

How will I be induced? Most obstetric units use a combination of methods to induce labour. To start with, your cervix needs to ripen (soften) and begin to dilate for labour to begin. If this has not happened naturally, you will be given a hormone called prostaglandin in the form of a gel or pessaries, which are inserted into your vagina so that the drug can work on your cervix. The advantage of this method is that it leaves you free to move around while the drug takes effect. Most units will keep you in hospital after administering prostaglandin, so that the midwife can regularly record the baby's heartbeat using a cardiotocograph (CTG) and monitor for signs of fetal distress.

If further measures are required, your midwife or doctor may perform an artificial rupture of membranes (ARM) – a painless procedure in which your waters are artificially broken, using a small tool not unlike a crochet hook. This removes the cushion of amniotic fluid between the baby's head and your cervix, encouraging labour to begin. You may also be given a drug called syntocinon, which mimics the natural hormone that stimulates contractions. Your baby's heartbeat will be monitored throughout the process.

Chapter 5

Medical emergencies

Medical emergencies only tend to happen in the **first and third trimesters**. Although these **tend to be rare**, it is wise to be **aware of the danger signs** so that you can seek medical help quickly if necessary.

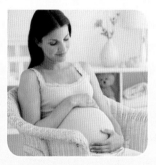
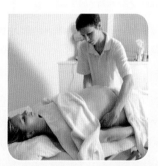
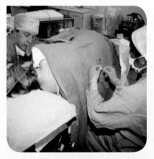

Vaginal bleeding

Vaginal bleeding at any stage of pregnancy should be taken seriously. It may indicate an abnormally placed placenta, known as placenta praevia (see p. 70), or it may be a warning of imminent miscarriage. Both of these conditions require prompt medical treatment.

Vaginal bleeding occurs in the first trimester in about a quarter of all pregnancies. Over half of these continue with delivery of a healthy baby at term. If vaginal bleeding occurs any time during the first three months:

✳ Call your doctor and he will arrange for you to have a scan in your local early pregnancy unit as soon as possible.

✳ If you pass any clots, mention this to your doctor, who may want to examine them.

✳ Don't take any medicine or drink any alcohol.

Emergency conditions

The vast majority of pregnancies continue to term with no problems or emergencies. However, it is sensible to make yourself aware of the danger signs so that you know when to seek professional medical attention.

Miscarriage

Medically known as spontaneous abortion, miscarriage is when the fetus delivers before the 24th week. After the 24th week, it is called a premature delivery or stillbirth. About a quarter of all pregnancies end in early miscarriage. Many occur before pregnancy has been confirmed or even suspected, so women are often unaware that they have miscarried, believing that they have only had a heavy period.

Miscarriage increases in frequency with age and with the number of previous pregnancies. They usually happen during the first trimester, the most common symptom being bleeding, which occurs in 95 per cent of cases. If bleeding occurs at any time in your pregnancy, you must consult your doctor.

Most miscarriages happen because the fetus fails to implant securely in the uterine wall. Often in one-off miscarriages there are chromosomal problems with the pregnancy. Maternal causes of miscarriage include uterine abnormalities such as large fibroids, and hormonal imbalances. Some bacterial and viral infections can also cause miscarriage. Cervical incompetence (see p. 72) accounts for only one per cent of spontaneous abortions. Paternal factors include abnormal sperm. Miscarriages are divided into several types:

Threatened miscarriage Miscarriage is possible but not inevitable. There is vaginal bleeding and sometimes pain. This occurs in about 10 per cent of all pregnancies and it may be confused with the slight bleeding that can occur at the time of the first missed period.

Inevitable miscarriage Vaginal bleeding is accompanied by pain because the uterus is contracting. If there is also dilation of the cervix, the loss of the pregnancy is bound to occur.

Incomplete miscarriage This is the term for when miscarriage has occurred but some of the products of conception, such as the amniotic sac or the placenta, remain in the uterus.

Complete miscarriage The fetus and placenta are expelled and the uterus returns to its normal size. This can be confirmed by ultrasound examination.

Missed miscarriage Either the fetus itself never properly developed or it died very early on. The placenta may still be functioning and the lack of a fetus may only be diagnosed when you have a scan.

Recurrent miscarriage Miscarriage has occurred on three or more occasions, sometimes for different reasons and at different stages of pregnancy (see column, right).

Treatment If you are bleeding, go to bed and stay there until the bleeding ceases. In particular, do not engage in activities such as strenuous exercise or sexual intercourse. If the bleeding and pain subside, you are quite likely to go on to deliver a healthy baby.

   If miscarriage appears to be inevitable, there is very little doctors can do to prevent it. If an incomplete miscarriage occurs, you may need an operation to make sure the uterus is completely empty, but in many cases you will be advised to wait and allow your body to absorb any remaining products. If heavy bleeding occurs, an operation may still be necessary. The uterus will be cleaned out by a procedure called an ERPC (evacuation of retained products of conception) usually under general anaesthetic. Painkillers are given, along with drugs to stop the bleeding. If a lot of blood has been lost, a transfusion may be necessary.

   There is no urgency in treating a missed miscarriage, but if, after a time, a spontaneous miscarriage hasn't occurred, an ERPC will be carried out. If fetal death occurs later in pregnancy, prostaglandin pessaries or an oxytocin injection will be given to stimulate delivery.

   Recurrent miscarriages that have occurred because of cervical incompetence can be treated by running a "purse-string" suture round the cervix at the beginning of the next pregnancy to ensure competency (see p. 72).

   Other possible reasons for recurrent miscarriage are genetic or hormonal disorders or problems with blood clotting. Long-term infections, such as listeria, may sometimes cause repeated miscarriages, but these can be difficult to diagnose and treat. If you do miscarry, talking over your feelings about

Repeated miscarriages

Possible reasons for recurrent miscarriages include:

✳ Genetic or hormonal disorders, although these are rare.

✳ Long-term infections, such as listeria, which may sometimes cause repeated miscarriages, and can be difficult to diagnose and treat.

✳ Poor nutrition.

✳ Chronic disease, such as renal disease.

✳ Cervical incompetence (see p. 72).

✳ Problems with the development of the blood supply to the placenta; for example, some women have excess clotting of their blood, in which case aspirin and heparin may help.

✳ Physical causes, including growths in the uterus (particularly fibroids), or structural abnormalities such as a partial or complete septum, which is a partial or full partition of the uterus; these can usually be corrected by surgery.

Some women will repeatedly miscarry even though exhaustive tests reveal no specific cause. Recent research has shown that supportive care can increase the chances of a successful pregnancy.

Placenta praevia

If the placenta has implanted incorrectly, it can obstruct the baby's birth.

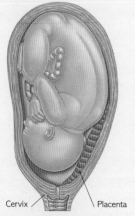

Cervix /   \ Placenta

Partial placenta praevia The placenta implants on the side and extends to the cervix, but does not cover it.

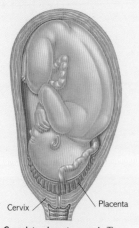

Cervix /   \ Placenta

Complete placenta praevia The placenta implants centrally, completely covering the cervix – even when the cervix is fully dilated.

losing the baby helps you both come to terms with your loss. Share your grief with your partner and close friends. Before trying to conceive again, wait for one normal menstrual period. It's only natural that the experience of a miscarriage may make you anxious about any future pregnancy. Eat well and get plenty of rest to allow your body to recuperate. When you do become pregnant again, make the most of your antenatal check-ups to answer any questions you may have about your pregnancy.

Placental separation

Bleeding can occur from the placenta as a result of the partial or complete separation of the placenta from the uterine wall. Blood builds up in the spaces and eventually escapes around the membranes and through the cervix into the vagina. Known as placental abruption (*abruptio placentae*), it occurs in about 1 in 200 pregnancies. The cause is unknown, but it tends to be more common in women who have had two or more children. Obstetricians divide placental separation into three types according to its severity:

In mild separation, blood loss can be slight. Bed-rest is the best treatment, with ultrasound examination to monitor the situation. If it occurs late in pregnancy, labour may be induced.

In moderate separation, a quarter of the placenta separates and 500 millilitres to 1 litre (between 1 and 2 pints) of blood is lost. This may require a blood transfusion and, if the baby is still alive, a Caesarean section is performed.

Severe separation is an acute emergency, when at least two-thirds of the placenta shears off the uterine wall, and 2 litres (4 pints) or more of blood is lost. This causes severe shock, disturbance of blood clotting, and kidney shutdown. A rapid blood transfusion will be given, and if the pregnancy is approaching term, a Caesarean section will be performed to save the baby. If placental abruption occurs before the third trimester, fetal death is inevitable.

Placenta praevia

This occurs when the placenta is implanted in the lower uterus instead of the upper part (see column, left). It therefore lies in front of the baby when she starts to descend the birth canal at the onset of labour. The baby cannot pass down the canal without dislodging the placenta, thereby interrupting her own blood supply. Placenta praevia is a major cause of bleeding after the 28th week. The cause is usually unknown.

The greater the proportion of the placenta lying in the lower part of the uterus, the greater the likelihood of complications during delivery. Even though the growth of the placenta slows down after the 30th week of pregnancy, the lower part of the uterus is increasing in length. Stress between the placenta and wall of the uterus may occur, leading to episodes of bleeding.

This extremely dangerous condition can be diagnosed well ahead of delivery by an ultrasound scan (see p. 32). Early symptoms include episodes of bleeding with bright red blood, which may occur after sexual intercourse. If this happens, the doctor will advise hospital admission for bed-rest, with a blood transfusion if necessary. Bed-rest should continue, if possible, until the 37th week, when the baby will be delivered by Caesarean section.

Postpartum haemorrhage is likely to occur after the delivery of the baby, and you'll be given drugs as soon as your baby is born to prevent this. In a very few cases, haemorrhage will continue despite treatment and then a hysterectomy may have to be considered. For these reasons, delivery in a well-equipped hospital where a blood transfusion service is on hand is vital.

Placental insufficiency

During pregnancy, the fetus receives oxygen and nourishment and excretes carbon dioxide and waste products via the umbilical cord and the placenta. A healthy placenta is therefore crucial in maintaining the health of the fetus. If the placenta fails to nourish your baby adequately, this is known as placental insufficiency.

Assessment and treatment Insufficiency may be indicated if you show less than normal weight gain, if your uterus is growing slowly, or if your baby's size on a scan is below average.

Ultrasound is the most reliable way to measure the growth of the baby. If it shows that the baby is not growing adequately, your doctor will carry out some extra tests. A bio-physical profile that takes account of fetal breathing, body movement and tone, and quantity of amniotic fluid may be compiled. A specialized ultrasound scan called a Doppler scan (see p. 34) will also be performed; this can tell doctors about the flow of blood through the placenta, indicating whether it is working properly. Placental insufficiency may warrant the induction of labour and possibly a Caesarean section.

Causes of insufficiency

The placenta may be unable to support the fetus adequately for a number of reasons:

* The placenta may have developed abnormally.

* The blood flow through the placenta may be restricted, or there might be a loss of placental tissue.

* The placenta may separate, or partly separate, from the uterine wall.

* The placenta may be too small or poorly developed.

* The pregnancy may go beyond the EDD, so that the ageing placenta no longer adequately supports the fetus.

* If the mother has diabetes, this can adversely affect the placenta.

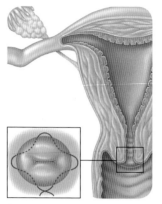

Suturing the cervix The cervix is kept closed by passing a suture right around it – like the strings of a purse. The stitch is normally removed about seven days before the expected date of delivery.

Incompetent cervix

During pregnancy, the cervix normally remains tightly shut and is sealed with a plug of mucus. This means that the fetus is safely held in the uterus until labour begins, when the cervix begins to dilate.

Occasionally, however, the cervical canal is incompetent and begins to open before term, usually in the third or fourth month. This allows the amniotic sac containing the fetus to sag through into the vagina, and possibly rupture, with a sudden loss of amniotic fluid followed by miscarriage. Unless the cervix has been damaged during previous surgery or pregnancy, this condition is fortunately rare. However, an incompetent cervix is usually diagnosed only after a first miscarriage has occurred.

If cervical incompetence is thought to be the cause of a previous miscarriage, treatment involves suturing your cervix, which means a soft non-absorbable thread is inserted in the cervix to keep it closed (see left). The stitch is removed approximately seven days before term, and your baby is delivered vaginally in the normal way.

Pre-eclampsia

Pregnancy-induced hypertension (high blood pressure), or pre-eclampsia, is a potentially dangerous condition that can affect as many as 1 in 10 women, especially first-time mothers and women carrying more than one baby. It is unique to pregnancy, starting at any time in the second half. It is not known what causes the condition, but it does tend to run in families. We do know that pre-eclampsia arises in the placenta, and so the baby may grow more slowly than normal.

Symptoms Pre-eclampsia is symptomless, but raised blood pressure and protein in the urine detected at an antenatal visit may alert staff to its presence.

Treatment A pregnancy complicated by pre-eclampsia cannot be restored to normal, but delivery of the baby and placenta ends the condition. Admission to hospital allows close monitoring of mother and baby so that delivery can be arranged before serious complications such as eclampsia (see p. 73) arise. For almost every mother, delivery of the baby reverses all the effects.

Eclampsia

The word eclampsia derives from the Greek words meaning "like a flash of lightning" because it seemed to strike out of the blue with fits, and eventually coma. Eclampsia is a potentially life-threatening condition for both mother and baby and it used to be quite common. However, it is now extremely rare in the West owing to the ability of doctors to diagnose the condition in its earliest phase (pre-eclampsia, see p. 72), and doctors and midwives are constantly alert for the warning signs. When eclampsia does occur, it is a full-blown medical emergency.

Symptoms Eclampsia is an emergency because the blood vessels in the uterus go into spasm (vasospasm), thereby cutting down the blood flow to the fetus with dangerously low levels of oxygen in the tissues (hypoxia).

The mother's life is threatened because vasospasm leads to kidney failure. Brain oxygen is also lowered, causing heightened brain sensitivity, which shows as fits. Tissues become waterlogged because of fluid retention, and haemorrhages can occur in tissues such as the liver. The earliest signs are drowsiness, headache, dimness of vision, all of which are superimposed on rising blood pressure, swelling of hands, face, and feet (oedema), and protein in the urine.

Treatment Where eclampsia develops, like pre-eclampsia, treatment is aimed at increasing blood flow to the brain, reducing high blood pressure, and delivering the baby – usually by Caesarean section. Within 24 hours of the baby being delivered, the condition subsides.

Ectopic pregnancy

In ectopic pregnancy, the fertilized egg implants somewhere other than in the cavity of the uterus, usually in the Fallopian tube. The rapidly growing embryo causes the tube to distend, and the invading placenta weakens its walls, causing bleeding. Eventually the tube bursts under the strain.

However, before this, certain symptoms that signal all is not well (see column, right) usually occur around the sixth week of pregnancy. Report any such symptoms to your doctor at once.

Types of ectopic pregnancy

Doctors define two forms of ectopic pregnancy:

Subacute This is signalled by pain in the abdomen, usually only on one side, sometimes with vaginal bleeding, fainting, and pain in the shoulder. It may not be detected until eight to 10 weeks' gestation. It is sometimes treatable by injecting a drug into the ectopic, causing it to die and be reabsorbed, which can save the Fallopian tube.

Acute form This happens when the tube bursts, leading to severe pain and shock, with extreme paleness, weak but rapid pulse, and falling blood pressure. A ruptured ectopic pregnancy requires immediate hospital admission and surgery.

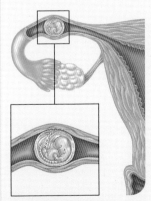

Tubal implantation Ectopic pregnancy occurs in about 1 in every 300 pregnancies. In 99 per cent of cases, the egg implants in the Fallopian tube. Very rarely, it may implant elsewhere.

Taking paternity leave

In Britain, there is now a provision for most fathers-to-be and long-term partners of expectant mothers to take paternity leave.

You can choose to take one or two weeks of leave, which must be taken all together. (You can't take odd days here and there.)

To qualify for paid paternity leave, you must be the father of the child, the husband or partner of the mother, or the adopter or partner of the adopter of the child. You must also be in contracted employment, and have been with the company for a minimum length of time. These rules also apply to women in same-sex relationships.

If you do not meet these conditions, you can still take some time off, either as unpaid leave agreed with your employer, or as part of your paid holiday for the year.

Your rights

Pregnant women are entitled to certain rights and benefits depending on their circumstances and national insurance contributions. The entitlements, particularly for those on low incomes, are complicated but any Social Security office or Citizens' Advice Bureau will be able to work out what you can claim. If you are employed, ask your employer or your trade union representative about your maternity leave and pay.

State benefits

The Maternity Allowance is a tax-free allowance you may receive if you can't get Statutory Maternity Pay (see right) because you have recently stopped working, changed jobs, or become self-employed. It is paid for a maximum of 39 weeks and is dependent on your national insurance contributions.

If you or your partner are receiving Income Support, Jobseeker's Allowance, Family Credit, or Disability Allowance, you may be able to get a cash payment (called a Maternity Payment) from the Social Fund. The rules are explained in leaflets that you can get from your local Social Security office, Citizens Advice Bureau, or antenatal clinic.

During your pregnancy and for one year after the birth you are eligible for free prescriptions and dental treatment, and you may get free milk if you are on a low income. You may also be eligible for Child Benefit, a Child Trust Fund, and possibly Child Tax Credits.

Working women

It is the law in Great Britain that your job must be kept open for you for a period of 52 weeks, starting from 11 weeks prior to your expected date of delivery, no matter how long you have been with your employer or how many hours you work for them. This consists of 26 weeks Ordinary Maternity Leave (OML), followed by 26 weeks of Additional Maternity Leave (AML). After OML, you are entitled to return to your job. After AML, you are entitled to return to your job, or to a similar job under similar terms and conditions.

Discuss all aspects and conditions with your employer and make it clear whether you wish to return to work so that your job will be kept open for you. Your employer may have more generous maternity pay and leave entitlements than those provided by law. As long as you have been employed by that employer since before you became pregnant and are earning enough per week (before tax) to pay National Insurance contributions, you should receive Statutory Maternity Pay (SMP) from your employer during the first 39 weeks of leave. They can claim this back from the government. You don't have to be intending to return to work to receive SMP.

While pregnant you are also entitled to paid time off for antenatal care, and you're protected against unfair dismissal. Working out your exact entitlement may seem daunting, but you can get help from your employer's human resources department and from independent organizations such as the Citizens' Advice Bureau and your trade union.

Work hazards

If your job is dangerous or it would be illegal for you to continue doing it, for example, if you work with anaesthetic gases or toxic chemicals, your employer must find you an alternative job or transfer you to a non-hazardous working place.

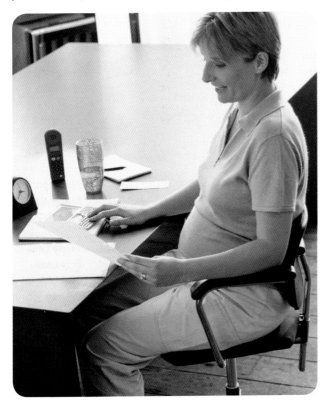

When to give up work When to stop working is entirely your decision. Most women stop work at 34 or 36 weeks, but you might be advised by your doctor to stop working if you have a pregnancy-related illness, a medical problem, or if you are expecting twins, as the strain might prove too much.

Claiming your rights

The chart below gives you a timetable for claiming benefits and notifying your employer, so that you can be sure of getting your maximum entitlement in terms of money and rights.

Rights and benefits timetable

WHEN	WHAT TO DO	WHY
As soon as you know you are pregnant	1 Ask doctor or midwife for form FW8 2 Tell your dentist (if you need treatment) 3 Check leaflet HC11 and tell Social Security office if you are getting Income Support 4 Tell your employer 5 Find out if you can get Maternity Allowance	1 To apply for free prescriptions 2 To apply for free dental treatment 3 To check your right to free spectacles, and help with hospital fares 4 To check whether you can get SMP (Statutory Maternity Pay) and for right to paid time off for antenatal visits 5 If you can't get SMP
As soon as you can	If you are unemployed or sick, check with Social Security office about Maternity Allowance claim	It can affect the amount of Maternity Allowance you may get
At least three weeks before you intend to stop working	Tell your employer in writing: the date you will stop working, when the baby is due, and whether you intend to return to your job	To protect your rights to SMP, and to return to work
As soon after the birth as you can	1 Register baby's birth 2 Send off form for Child Benefit and Family Premium if you are a single parent 3 Check low income benefits	1 To get the birth certificate 2 To get Child Benefit and Lone Parent payment 3 To see if you qualify for Maternity Payment from Social Fund, and spectacles, milk and vitamins, hospital fares, and help with your rent and council tax
Three weeks after birth or	Register baby (if you live in Scotland)	Latest date to do this
Six weeks after birth	Register baby (England, Wales, and Ireland)	Latest date to do this
Eight weeks before returning to work	Write to your employer stating the date that you wish to return	To protect your right to return to work
52 weeks after the start of your maternity leave	Latest date by which you have a right to go back to your job	You may lose your right to return to work

Useful addresses

Active Birth Centre
25 Bickerton Road
London N19 5JT
Tel: 020 7281 6760
www.activebirthcentre.com
Information and classes on active involvement in childbirth at home or in hospital

AIMS (Association for Improvements in Maternity Services)
5 Ann's Court
Grove Road, Surbiton
Surrey KT6 4BE
Tel: 020 300 365 0663
www.aims.org.uk
Pressure group that campaigns for the right of parents to have the maternity services they want

APEC (Action on Pre-eclampsia)
2c The Halfcroft
Syston LE7 1LD
Tel: 020 8427 4217
www.apec.org.uk

Association of Breastfeeding Mothers
PO Box 207, Bridgewater
TA6 7YT
Tel: 08444 122 949
www.abm.me.uk
A 24-hour telephone service for mothers. Supplies nationwide network of breastfeeding counsellors

Birthworks
58 Malpas Road
Brockley
London SE4 1BS
Tel: 0333 240 9710
www.birthworks.co.uk
Advice and literature on water births, birth pools for hire

BLISS (Baby Life Support Systems)
9 Holyrood Street
London SE1 2EL
Tel: 0500 618 140
www.bliss.org.uk
Advice and support for parents with special-care babies

British Acupuncture Council
63 Jeddo Road
London W12 9HQ
Tel: 020 8735 0400
www.acupuncture.org.uk

British Epilepsy Association
New Anstey House
Gate Way Drive
Yeadon, Leeds LS19 7XY
Tel: 01132 108800
www.epilepsy.org.uk

Diabetes UK
Macleod House
10 Parkway, London NW1 7AA
Tel: 020 7424 1000
www.diabetes.org.uk
Advice for pregnant women with diabetes

Down's Syndrome Association
Langdon Down Centre, 2a Langdon
Park, Teddington TW11 9PS
Tel: 0845 230 0372
www.downs-syndrome.org.uk
Advice on the care of children with Down's syndrome

Freeline Social Security Number
0800 882200
Free helpline for information about maternity benefits

Independent Midwives' Association
PO Box 539
Abingdon OX14 9DF
Tel: 0845 4600 105
www.independentmidwives.org.uk
Network of independent midwives offering private care

Maternity Action
Tindlemanor
52-53 Featherstone Street
London EC1Y 8RT
Tel: 020 7253 2288
www.maternityaction.org.uk
Information on maternity rights and benefits

Miscarriage Association
c/o Clayton Hospital, Northgate
Wakefield
West Yorkshire WF1 3JS
Tel: 01924 200 799
www.miscarriageassociation.org.uk

MS Therapy Centres
7 Peartree Business Centre
Peartree Road
Stanway, Colchester
Essex CO3 0JN
Tel: 0800 783 0518
www.msrc.co.uk
Information for pregnant women suffering from MS

National Childbirth Trust
Alexandra House
Oldham Terrace
London W3 6NH
Tel: 0870 770 3236
www.nctpregnancyandbabycare.com
For antenatal classes and postnatal help

RCOG (Royal College of Obstetricians and Gynaecologists)
27 Sussex Place
Regent's Park
London NW1 4RG
Tel: 020 7772 6200
www.rcog.org.uk

Royal College of Midwives
15 Mansfield Street
London W1G 9NH
www.rcm.org.uk
Tel: 020 7312 3535

TAMBA (Twins and Multiple Birth Association)
2 The Willows
Gardner Road
Guildford
Surrey GU1 4PG
Tel: 0800 138 0509
www.tamba.org.uk
Offers encouragement and support for parents before and after multiple births

Vegetarian Society
Parkdale Dunham Road
Altrincham
Cheshire WA14 4QG
Tel: 0161 925 2000
www.vegsoc.org
Nutritional advice for pregnant women who are vegetarians

Women's Health
www.womens-health.co.uk
Advice on reproductive health

Index

A

abortion, spontaneous, 68–69
age, effect of, 60, 61
alpha-fetoprotein (AFP), 31, 57, 60
amenorrhoea, 8
amniocentesis, 14, 31, 57–58, 60, 62
amniotic fluid, 28, 56, 57
anaemia, 20, 27, 31
ankles, swollen, 17, 26
anomaly scan, 34
antenatal care, 13, 15, 17, 24–25
antenatal clinics, 24
antenatal tests, 26–31
anti-D injection, 62
appetite, 12, 13, 18
artificial rupture of
  membranes (ARM), 66

B

baby's arrival, preparing for, 17
backache, 15, 16
bilirubin, 58, 62, 63
birth plan, 52–54
birthing rooms, 43, 44
bleeding, vaginal, 68–71
blood group, 30
blood pressure, 17, 29, 72
blood tests, 9, 27, 29, 30–31
body, changes to, 12, 13, 14
bras, maternity, 12, 13
Braxton Hicks' contractions, 17
breasts:
  breast shields, 26
  changes in, 9, 12
  examination of, 26
breathing, 16, 48–49
breech presentation, 24

C

calcium, 20
carbohydrates, 13, 18, 19
carers, professional, 22–23
  talking to, 24

cervical incompetence, 68–69, 72
childbirth, choices in, 38–39
childbirth classes, 46–47
  childbirth teachers, 47
  father's role in, 47
chorionic villus sampling (CVS), 56–57
chromosomal defects, 60, 61
clothes:
  for baby, 17
  for mother, 13
cognitive control, 47
colostrum, 14
conception, 8
confirming pregnancy, 9
  home testing, 10–11
constipation, 14, 17
consultant obstetricians, 22
contractions, 44, 45, 66
  Braxton Hicks', 17
  early in pregnancy, 29
cordocentesis, 31, 59, 62, 63
cravings, food, 9
cystic fibrosis, 57

D

dental care, 14
diabetes, 27, 31
diet, 12–13, 18–20
  daily requirements, 18
  eating for two, 18
  food cravings, 9
  for vegetarians, 20
  nutrition, 13, 18–20
  preparing food, 20
  to avoid, 20
digestion, problems in, 14
Doppler scan, 34, 61
Down's syndrome:
  age, effect of, 60
  amniocentesis, 57–58
  chorionic villus sampling (CVS), 56–57
  nuchal scan, 31, 34, 60
  triple test, 30, 31, 60

E

eclampsia, 73
ectopic pregnancy, 73
Edward's syndrome, 58
electronic fetal monitoring, 65
emergencies, 68–73
engagement, 16
Entonox, 45
episiotomy, 41
estimated date of delivery
  (EDD), 11, 64, 65
exercise:
  classes, 47
  during pregnancy, 50–51
external examination, 28

F

fathers:
  paternity leave, 74
  role in childbirth classes, 47
fetal anaemia, 59
fetal heart monitoring, 29, 61
fetal movement recording, 65
first trimester, 12–13
fluid retention, 26
folic acid, 19, 27
food:
  see diet
fundus, 28

G

general practitioner (GP), 22
German measles:
  see rubella
glucose tolerance test, 31
growth restriction, fetal, 59
gums, 14

H

haemoglobin:
  blood tests, 27, 30
  chorionic villus sampling (CVS), 56–57

electrophoresis test, 31
haemophilia, 57, 58
hands, swollen, 17, 26
Hawthorne rehearsal, 47
heartbeat, fetal, 29, 61, 66
heartburn, 14
height, 26
hepatitis B, 30
high-tech birth, 38, 39
HIV test, 31
home birth, 39, 40
  preparing for, 44–45
hormones, 8, 10, 12, 15
hospital birth, 38, 41
  choosing a hospital, 42–43
  natural birthing units, 43
hospital midwives, 23
human chorionic gonadotrophin
  (hCG), 9, 10, 30, 60
Huntington's chorea, 57
hypnobirthing, 47
hypoxia, 73
hysterectomy, 71

I
incompetent cervix, 68–69, 72
independent midwives, 23
inducing labour, 65–66
internal examination, 28–29
iron, 18, 19, 20, 27, 30
ischaemia, 64

K, L
ketones, 27
labour:
  anxiety about, 16
  preparation for, 48–49
legs, examination of, 26
lie of the baby, 25
linea nigra, 15
listeria, 20
lovemaking, 17
lymphocytes, fetal, 59

M
managed birth, 38–39
massage, 17
maternity bras, 12, 13
maternity leave, 74
medical terminology, 25
metabolism, rate of, 12
midwives, 23, 40, 44, 45
minerals, 20
miscarriage, 68–69
Montgomery's tubercles, 12
mood changes, 12
morning sickness, 9, 19, 26
muscular dystrophy, 57, 58

N
natural birth, 36, 39
nausea, 26
nipples:
  changes in, 12, 14
  examination of, 26
nuchal scan, 31, 34, 60
nutrition, 13, 18–20

O
obstetricians, consultant, 22, 52
oedema, 26, 73
oestriol, 60
oestrogen, 12
overdue babies, 64–66

P
pain, coping with, 47
  pain relief philosophies, 36–37
panting, 49
Patau's syndrome, 58
paternity leave, 74
pelvic disproportion, 27
pelvic floor exercises, 48
periods, missing, 8
pethidine, 45
philosophies, childbirth, 36–37
pigmentation, 15

placenta, 64, 70–71
  abruption, 70
  insufficiency, 64, 71
  separation, 70
  placenta praevia, 68, 69, 70–71
post-mature babies, 64–65
postpartum haemorrhage, 71
posture, 15
pre-eclampsia, 26, 27, 29, 72
pregnancy tests, 9–11
progesterone, 8, 12, 48
prostaglandin, 66, 69
proteins, 13, 18, 19

R
relaxation, 16, 17, 49
results, of home pregnancy tests, 10–11
Rhesus incompatibility, 27, 30,
  58, 62–63
rights and benefits, 74–76
rubella, 30, 59

S
salmonella, 20
second trimester, 14–15
sex, baby's, 57
shoe size, 26
sickle-cell disease, 31, 56
signs of pregnancy, 8–9, 13
sleep, 16–17
smell, sense of, 9
Sonicaid, 29, 40, 45, 61
specialized scans, 34
special tests, 56–61
sphygmomanometer, 45
spontaneous abortion, 68–69
state benefits, 74–75
stillbirth, 65
swelling, of ankles, 17, 26
syntocinon, 41, 66
syntometrine, 45
syphilis, 30
systematic relaxation, 47

T

tastes, odd, 9

team midwives, 23

tests:

  antenatal, 26–31

  for pregnancy, 9–11

    precautions, 10

  special tests, 56–61

thalassaemia, 31, 57

third trimester, 16–17

tiredness, 8, 16, 17

toxoplasmosis, 20, 30, 59

trimesters:

  first, 12–13

  second, 14–15

  third, 16–17

  triple test, 30, 31, 60

U

ultrasound scanning, 15, 29, 32–34, 60

umbilical vein sampling, 59

urination, frequent, 8, 13, 17

urine tests, 9–11, 17, 27

uterus, 12, 13, 14

V

vaginal bleeding, 68–71

varicose veins, 26

vasospasm, 73

vegetarian diet, 20

vitamins, 18, 19

W, X

weight gain, 15, 18, 19, 26

work hazards, during pregnancy, 75

X-ray, 33

Acknowledgments

The publisher would like to thank the following for their kind permission to reproduce their photographs:

(Key: a-above; b-below/bottom; c-centre; l-left; r-right; t-top)

2 Corbis: Jose Luis Pelaez, Inc. / Blend Images. 5 Corbis: Larry Williams (cra). Getty Images: Blend Images / ERproductions Ltd (br); Paul Bradbury (tr); John Lund (crb). 8 Getty Images: Paul Bradbury. 27 Mother & Baby Picture Library: Ian Hooton. 32 Mother & Baby Picture Library: Ian Hooton. 33 Science Photo Library. 34 Science Photo Library. 35 Getty Images: Thomas Northcut (br). 55 Getty Images: Tom Grill (bc). 61 Science Photo Library: Ian Hooton. 67 Getty Images: Ben Edwards (br); Tetra Images (bl)

Jacket images: Front: Getty Images: JGI/Jamie Grill. Back: Getty Images: Adam Gault/SPL

DK would like to thank
UK medical consultant: Dr Elizabeth Owen
Proofreader: Angela Baynham

All other images © Dorling Kindersley
For further information see:
www.dkimages.com